Canine Epilepsy
& Seizures

Canine Epilepsy & Seizures

Causes and Treatments

James Belan

Copyright © 2018 by James Belan.

ISBN: Hardcover   978-1-9845-5048-4
         Softcover   978-1-9845-5047-7
         eBook   978-1-9845-5046-0

All rights reserved. No part of this book may be reproduced or transmitted in any form or by any means, electronic or mechanical, including photocopying, recording, or by any information storage and retrieval system, without permission in writing from the copyright owner.

The views expressed in this work are solely those of the author and do not necessarily reflect the views of the publisher, and the publisher hereby disclaims any responsibility for them.

Any people depicted in stock imagery provided by Getty Images are models, and such images are being used for illustrative purposes only.
Certain stock imagery © Getty Images.

Print information available on the last page.

Rev. date: 09/14/2018

To order additional copies of this book, contact:
Xlibris
1-888-795-4274
www.Xlibris.com
Orders@Xlibris.com
773804

DEDICATION

This book is dedicated to my wife, Lorri Belan, who unselfishly gave her time to care for our yellow lab who began having seizures when he was eighteen months old. Her passion was to find a cure for our dog Chowder, spending countless hours looking for answers. This included scouring the Internet canine world and joining as many online canine epilepsy fora that were available to gain as much knowledge as possible and hope that the next e-mail or article she read would bring her hope for her best friend Chowder. Her quest gave me the inspiration to get as much information and knowledge to help other dog owners who love their dogs as much as we loved ours. This information may help you cope with this malady and maybe find your cure.

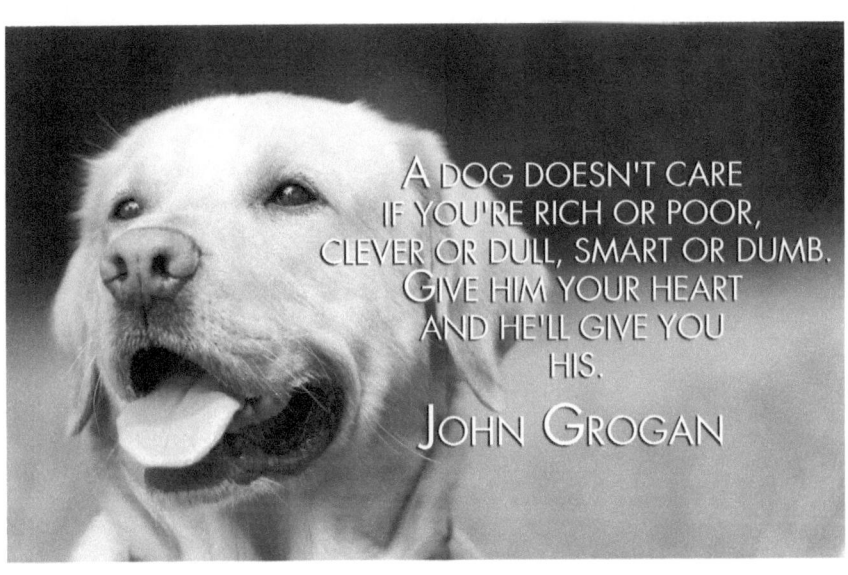

Contents

Dedication v
Preface xi

PART I
SEIZURES

Chapter 1   What Is a Seizure? 1
Chapter 2   What Is Canine Epilepsy? 9
Chapter 3   Types of Seizures (or Epilepsy in Dogs) 11
Chapter 4   When a Seizure Occurs 17
Chapter 5   What Happens During a Seizure 19
Chapter 6   What to Do When Your Dog Is Having a Seizure 21
Chapter 7   Care After a Seizure 29
Chapter 8   Diagnoses for Dog Seizures 34

PART II
CAUSES OF SEIZURES

Introduction to the Causes of Seizures 39
Chapter 9   Disease 41
Chapter 10   Chemicals 45
Chapter 11   Medical Conditions 48
Chapter 12   The Thyroid 61
Chapter 13   Genetics 64
Chapter 14   Mycotoxins 67
Chapter 15   Diet, Nutrition, and Seizures 71
Chapter 16   Heatstroke 84
Chapter 17   Vaccines 88
Chapter 18   Flea and Tick Prevention 94

Chapter 19 Medications and Drugs 101
Chapter 20 What Foods Are Toxic to Dogs 107
Chapter 21 Plants 114
Chapter 22 What is the Immune System? 148
Chapter 23 Yard and Garden 155
Chapter 24 Dog Collars 168
Chapter 25 Stress 169
Chapter 26 The Household 171

PART III
TREATMENTS FOR SEIZURE

Introduction to the Treatment of Seizures 183
Chapter 27 Seizure Medications 185
Chapter 28 The Liver 201
Chapter 29 Treatment with Diet 209
Chapter 30 Natural, Homeopathic, and Holistic Treatment 220
Chapter 31 Treatment of Status Epilepsy 234

PART IV
THE CAREGIVER & PROGNOSIS

Chapter 32 The Caregiver 238
Chapter 33 Prognosis 242

PREFACE

The story that made this book a reality began in the summer of 2004, while I was working in Kennewick, Washington, on a construction project with a good friend of mine, Dan Lopez. He asked me to look in on his beautiful female white Labrador, Sierra, who was pregnant and ready to give birth any day. Being a car enthusiast, he had plans for that day at a car show some 100 miles away. I was glad to look in on Sierra since she had a great personality and was a very friendly white lab. I drove over to his place and let Sierra out to the backyard to relieve herself and get some exercise by throwing the tennis ball for her. It was not long before she dug a shallow hole under a bush and started to give birth. So much for the spot prepared in the garage with old blankets. She quickly had six tiny bundles, which she licked clean and doted over. I called Dan, my buddy, at the car show and gave him the news. "Dan, you have six new puppies!" I exclaimed. "Okay, great, I'll be home after the show. See ya soon." Two minutes later, Sierra had two more puppies. Five minutes later, two more puppies came for a total of ten. Sierra came to me in the back yard after she cleaned the pups, with the tennis ball in her mouth, and wanted me to throw the ball, something she would do all day long if you let her. I took the ball and she backed away, anticipating my throw, then she stopped and right there in the middle of the back yard she squatted and out came the last puppy, the runt of the litter. (This guy turned out to be my buddy, Chowder.) She gently picked the tiny bundle up in her mouth and went to her nest under the bush and placed the last pup. I called Dan and told him the news: He had eleven new labs, seven chocolate and four white, and he said he will be right home. Not being a midwife for a dog before, I called my wife and asked for advice on what was required for newborn puppies. She gave me instructions on building a wilting box to keep the pups safe so I went to the local lumber store and built a box. Now I needed to get the pups into the garage. Since Sierra was very protective of her brood, I devised a plan to get her into the house and close the door behind her. I called her and she came and in she went with the door closing behind her. Now I had time to move the precious cargo into the garage into the new box I had made. I first cleaned each one of the sand clinging to them from the shallow pit mom had made. Then they were placed on the old bed spread in the box safely in the garage. Opening the door, Sierra started for the back door before I called her attention to the box and her pups. She immediately went over and settled in and started to feed her little ones. Dan had gotten home with his wife, and they were excited over their new family. At that time he offered me pick of the litter.

I was awed by the offer. I really loved Sierra, and I thought that a white lab like her would be great, so my choice was one of the four white/yellow pups, which included the runt. Something about him drew me to him. Sometimes you just know. Anyway after four weeks and the project was over and with his eyes open, I hopped into my pickup with the puppy with no name and we headed to my home in Arizona. The first stop, though, was the Portland airport to pick up my wife who flew in for a mini vacation trip home along the beautiful coast of Oregon and California. I introduced her to my lil buddy, and leaving the Portland airport, we started our trip along the Oregon coast, starting at Lincoln City. We stopped for lunch at a seafood place called Moe's, and we got each a bowl of their famous clam chowder. We got it to go and sat in the truck and ate so we could stay with the pup-with-no-name. He was beside himself trying to get a taste of the chowder from us. With a bit on the tip of a spoon, he practically chewed the spoon. Our new puppy got his name: Chowder. He even had the same coloring as clam chowder. On the trip home he slept between us in the truck or in a hotel bed.

Luckily, he could fit in my jacket pocket with no problem when we would sneak him pass the hotel desk.

Chowder was smart as he was cute. At a training class, he won the prize as the most improved and intelligent dog in the class. At our home in Arizona, we had a pool with a sloping concrete ramp at the water line so the dogs (we had another cocker) could get in and out of the water and also the birds and small wildlife critters can get a drink of water. Chowder loved the water. Whenever we threw in a tennis ball into the pool, he would go airborne as gracefully as an Olympic diver and retrieve it, begging for you to throw it again.

Then ours, and his world turned for the worst.

We came home one day from shopping and a flower pot was on its side without explanation. This never happened before, and it was a mystery to us. Then a few weeks later I was in the back yard with my two dogs, Sophie, my cocker, and Chowder, my yellow lab. Chowder was standing around me as I was doing some yard work, and it happened. He stiffened up, yelped, and started off running in a semicircle, only to collapse in a garden bed and go into convulsions. His legs were straight out shaking, and his teeth were clacking together with lips pulled back and he had this wild look in his eyes. I was stunned. I did not know what to do. My cocker spaniel went up to him and was sniffing him as he was shuttering uncontrollable. I knew I was witnessing a canine seizure but had no idea what to do. After a short, period he loosened up and it was over. He was dazed as if just coming out of unconsciousness, so I gave him some time and he got up after a while and came over to me as if to ask what happened. He licked my hand as he always did, and I held him tight, hoping I never see that again. Unfortunately it was just the beginning of the nightmare that was to come for the rest of my lil buddy's life.

After that seizure, we rushed him to the vet to get a diagnosis. The vet listened to what we witnessed and explained canine epilepsy and seizure to us with a prognosis. If we cannot find the root cause of the seizure, he may get progressively worse with a poor quality of life and eventually shorten his life. That night I went on the Internet to find out all I can about a cure for my companion. Unfortunately there is not a lot available, but I wrote down everything I could and hoped for news of a wonder drug or treatment. The veterinarian medical world knows little to nothing about stopping seizures and only can curb it some in some dogs with drugs. In our case the drugs did little to stem the seizures, but only made him lethargic and listless. Thus, began the search for a cure that lasted until he could no longer fight the fight. At nine years and two months, Chowder went out in the morning to relieve himself and crossed the rainbow bridge. It was August 13, 2013. The most loving dog I ever knew. Rest in peace, my good buddy,

PART I

SEIZURES

Chapter 1

What Is a Seizure?

Seizures are one of the most common neurological conditions in dogs. The scientific term for seizure is "ictus." A seizure may also be called a convulsion, attack, or fit and is a temporary involuntary disturbance of normal brain function that is usually accompanied by uncontrollable muscle activity. They occur when too much electrical activity is going on in the outer layers of a dog's brain, called the "cortex," which is responsible for thought, memory, sensation, and movement. Seizures are the result of muscle responses to an abnormal nerve-signal burst from the brain. They are a symptom of an underlying neurological dysfunction. Toxic substances, metabolic or electrolyte abnormalities, and/or imbalances cause an uncoordinated firing of neurons in the cerebrum of the brain, creating seizures from mild "petit mal" to severe "grand mal." Seizures can be caused by many things, including infections, cancer, abscesses, anatomical malformations, heat stroke, liver disease, kidney disease, trauma, ingestion of toxins, and others, which will be addressed later on in this book. Neurons in a dog's brain communicate with each other through electrical and chemical signals that will either excite or shut down a neuron. When a dog's brain function is normal, the turning off and on of neurons is well balanced. But when too many neurons are turned on, a seizure occurs. Many times a dog that has a seizure is at rest or asleep, but some dogs can have a seizure after being stressed out.

The scientific term for seizure is "ictus" and the convulsion is caused by a temporary, involuntary disturbance of brain activity A seizure begins unexpectedly and ends suddenly and does occur again. Seizures typically last less than two minutes. They are characterized by stiff extended legs, collapse, breathing lapses, rhythmic leg jerking, chomping, drooling, and sometimes urination or defecation. As the uncontrolled discharge of neurons in the brain spreads, a partial seizure can become a generalized seizure. A generalized or grand mal is the most common form of a seizure. It is interesting to note that "mal," meaning bad or wrong or ill, is generally used as a prefix, for example "maladroit" (bungling). Seizures come in two types: primary and secondary. Some external influence or some outside stimulus causes secondary seizures. Primary epilepsy, also known by the names of idiopathic or genetic or inherited or true epilepsy, has no known source. With secondary seizures, the source is known.

The seizure itself is broken into four phases.

- Prodrome phase
- Pre-ictal, or sometimes called the aura phase
- Ictal phase – Ictal is from the Latin *ictus*, meaning attack
- Post-ictal

The Prodrome Phase (Pre-Ictus)

The pre-seizure phase causes behavioral changes and can begin more than twenty-four hours before an actual seizure and may last for minutes to hours. You may notice a subtle change in the behavior of your dog. The dog may be aware that something is wrong and will appear restless, pace, seek affection, salivate, whine, or hide. The dog may seek out affection or hide from the owner. In medicine, a prodrome is an early symptom (or set of symptoms) that might indicate the start of a disease before specific symptoms occur. It is derived from the Greek word *prodromos*, meaning "precursor."

The Aura (Intense Pre-Ictal or Focal Onset Phase)

The aura (intense pre-iIctus or focal onset) is when the conditions that occur in the prodome are intensified, and the dog experiences an altered state or a change in behavior. This may include altered emotions, visual perceptions, hearing, smelling, or tasting. In this stage just before the ictus (scizure), the dog may appear restless, with twitching and nervousness. The warning signs are a change in your dog's behavior. Prior to the seizure, your dog may have the following signs:

- Staring into space (faraway look)
- Drooling
- Agitation
- Nervousness
- Confusion
- Restlessness
- Seek affection or attention seeking
- Tries to hide or seeks seclusion
- Barking or howl (vocalization)

The pre-ictal phase is characterized by an obvious change in your dog's behavior (it may seem that the canine understands something is about to occur). Many dogs intensify the conditions of the prodome phase and the dog experiences an altered state or change in behavior. This may include altered emotions, visual perceptions, hearing, smelling, or tasting. In this stage just before the ictus (seizure), the dog may appear restless, with twitching, nervousness, and become anxious before a seizure. Just like humans, dogs often get warning signs when a seizure is coming. The warning comes in the form of an aura, not unlike the kind of aura humans with migraines and other neurological disturbances experience. Animals have a "sixth sense" about certain upcoming events, and canine epilepsy is one of them.

They can be confusing and can be a source of panic for your pet. You may see your dog go through the following changes as he experiences a seizure. Your dog may seek you out for affection or may go into seclusion and hide, but either way will look frightened. Your dog may whine or shake as the seizure begins. Your dog's aura will typically make him or her feel and act scared, dazed, or worried. Your pet may also experience muscle and limb contractions, visual disturbances, and even loss of bowel and bladder control. A dog with seizures can also enter into a kind of altered mental status before a seizure hits, so be on the lookout for this and other neurological symptoms.

Before a dog has a tonic-clonic seizure, he will begin to feel dizzy or light-headed and may not be able to see or hear well. He may also act strange, upset, or nervous, and will begin repeating motions and may hide or demand his owner's attention. These symptoms are done in the aura (pre-ictal) phase. These actions occur because the seizure is beginning in one area of the dog's brain, the focus, which will eventually spread to the whole brain. The pre-ictal (aura phase) can last a few minutes up to a couple of hours.

The aura lasts from a few seconds to a few minutes before the ictus or actual seizure.

The Ictal Phase (The Seizure)

The ictal phase is the period during which the actual seizure occurs is the which usually lasts between a few seconds and five minutes. In a seizure, the dog will lose consciousness, will paddle or go through running movements, will chomp at the air and will salivate. Other symptoms of seizures may appear startling and even violent. They do not cause your dog pain. Dogs in an episode of convulsions will typically fall on their side, and their legs will jerk slightly or with a fair amount of force. Salivation or excessive drooling will take place. Your pet may urinate or defecate, and your dog's eyes may stare straight ahead. A severe episode may see a dog lose consciousness. If the seizure lasts more than five minutes, the dog must be taken to a veterinarian or animal medical hospital for professional medical treatment. As the seizure is ending, your dog may appear dazed and disoriented. Your pet may be uncoordinated. Temporary blindness may be experienced. Some dogs are restless, while others are fatigued. There may be increased thirst. Seizures occur because of uncontrolled, abnormal activity in the brain. Having seizures can be frightening for your pet because he loses control of his body. Muscle and brain function are impaired. The ictal phase is when a dog has the actual seizure. The "tonic" part of the seizure occurs when a dog's muscles become rigid, causing the canine to fall over with his legs sticking straight out and his head tilted back. This episode lasts about thirty seconds before the seizing begins. Signs a dog is in the ictal phase include the loss of consciousness, the twitching of muscles, and some involuntary vocalizations. The dog's eyes may remain open during a seizure, but he won't be able to see anything. A dog won't be able to control his bodily functions at this time and it's not usual for a canine to drool, urinate, empty his anal glands, and even defecate. The "clonic" phase of the seizure is when a dog unconsciously begins moving rhythmically. He may look like he is chomping on a big invisible bone or is running while lying down. A dog's tongue may also turn blue as he is not able to breathe well. This will typically last a couple of minutes. Rarely does a dog become vicious during a seizure. In fact, most dogs will actually feel the seizure coming on and seek out the owner for comfort. During the actual seizure, a dog is unaware of his surroundings so it does little good for the owner to try to comfort the seizuring dog. It is best to be there for comfort when the dog recovers.

The Post-Ictal Phase

The post-ictus is when the seizure is over and the dog appears to be dazed and confused. This can last from several minutes to several hours. Some dogs will pace around the house frantically like they are looking for something or walk in circles. Others will be temporarily blind and bump into walls. More than likely your dog will have to go outside to eliminate and after want a lot of fresh water. Since a seizure is traumatic to a dog's system and depletes it of glucose sugar in the blood, a couple spoons of ice cream or honey will restore the system to normal.

Note that in some dogs a seizure trigger could be a certain event, like poison to their system, low blood sugar, or a stressful condition. You will be able to recognize the conditions that cause a seizure by recognizing the common pattern (trigger) prior to the development of the event of a seizure. Was there smoke in the room? Loud noises like music? Something he ate in the yard? Did you treat the lawn with a weed killer, or use insecticide recently? By investigating and observation, you should recall if there is a possible trigger. There also may be a physical anomaly that would require a veterinarian visit to diagnose.

Seizures can happen when the dog is waking or falling asleep. Dogs who have seizures may appear normal otherwise. All dogs have a seizure threshold. A seizure occurs when this threshold is exceeded. Dogs with a low seizure threshold are divided into two groups: stimulus and nonstimulus. In the stimulus group, seizures may be caused by some external influence such as hormones, (e.g., estrogen, which can lower the threshold to seizures in parts of the brain), fatigue or injury, and hyperventilation. In the nonstimulus group, the seizures occur spontaneously. They have a sudden beginning. The nonstimulus seizure is typical of many idiopathic epileptic. Once the seizure is over, your dog may act as if nothing happened. But most post-seizure dogs will display altered behavioral characteristics for eighteen to twenty-four hours afterward. This includes confusion and disorientation as well as aimless wandering, compulsive behavior, momentary blindness, pacing, increased thirst, and even an increased appetite. Recovery may be immediate or take up to twenty-four hours.

Unfortunately, the number of seizures your dog has are linked to neuron damage in his or her brain. This in turn means your pet is more likely to experience seizures again. For research purposes, most experts classify all seizures in one of three ways:

1. Generalized seizures impact most of the brain and include both sides.
2. Focal seizures impact only a smaller, localized portion of the brain.
3. Focal seizures with secondary generalization are seizures that start out in one smaller place but then eventually lead to the rest of the brain seizing.

Convulsions, fits, or seizures cause the dog's body muscles to contract and relax rapidly. Although they are not typically life-threatening, the dog will lose control of its body, which can be frightening. In many cases, it is difficult to determine their underlying cause, but frequent recurrences are normally termed as *epilepsy*.

Is a Seizure Painful or Dangerous to the Dog?

Despite the dramatic and violent appearance of a seizure, seizures are not painful, although the dog may feel confusion and perhaps panic. Contrary to popular belief, dogs do not swallow their tongues during a seizure. If you put your fingers or an object into its mouth, you will not help your pet and you run a high risk of being bitten very badly or of injuring your dog. The important thing is to keep the dog from falling or hurting itself by knocking objects onto itself. As long as it is on the floor or ground, there is little chance of harm occurring.

A single seizure is rarely dangerous to the dog. However, if the dog has multiple seizures within a short period of time (cluster seizures), or if a seizure continues for longer than a few minutes, the body temperature begins to rise. If *hyperthermia* or an elevated body temperature develops secondary to a seizure, another set of problems may have to be addressed. As a general rule, younger dogs seem to have more severe epilepsy. When the onset is before the age of two, the condition will respond positively to medication. But the more seizures a dog has, the more likely there is to be damage among the neurons in the brain.

CHAPTER 2

What Is Canine Epilepsy?

Epilepsy affects around four in every hundred dogs. Canine epilepsy is used to describe repeated episodes of seizures. With epilepsy, the seizures can be single or may occur in clusters, and they can be infrequent and unpredictable or may occur at regular intervals. Canine epilepsy is a chronic condition characterized by recurring seizures. Seizures are described as an uncoordinated firing of the neurons usually within a portion of the brain called the *cerebrum*. The mechanisms of why these neurons do not function normally in epileptic dogs is not understood, but is similar if not identical to the causes in humans. Probably certain substances called *neurotransmitters* are not in the proper chemical balance.

Canine epilepsy is a disorder of the brain where abnormal electrical activity triggers further uncoordinated nerve transmission. This uncoordinated and haphazard nerve tissue activity scrambles messages to the muscles of your dog's body and the coordinated use of the muscles is then inhibited. Although seizures are always abnormal events, not all seizures in dogs are caused by canine epilepsy.

The term "epilepsy" is sometimes used interchangeably with "seizures," although technically this is not correct. Epileptic dogs do have unpredictable brain activity that causes them to have seizures, but not all dogs with seizures have epilepsy. There are many things that can cause a seizure in a dog. Epilepsy is just one of the many things that cause seizures. Just because a dog has a seizure does not mean that the dog has epilepsy. Because there are many causes of chronic recurrent seizures in dogs, canine epilepsy is not a specific disease or even a single syndrome, but rather a diverse category of disorders.

Canine epilepsy is broadly divided into idiopathic and symptomatic disorders. This will be discussed in chapter 3.

Chapter 3

Types of Seizures (or Epilepsy in Dogs)

Generalized seizures affect the whole body and can be divided into two types: grand mal and petit mal. Grand mal seizures are the most common. A dog experiencing a grand mal seizure usually falls on her side and has uncontrollable muscle activity such as kicking her legs as if swimming or paddling. Salivation is profuse and often the dog involuntarily urinates and defecates. The dog is unaware of you, her surroundings, or her own actions. Petit mal seizures do not result in convulsions, but the animal loses consciousness. It may look like the dog just collapsed.

The worst form of seizure is one in which the dog has one or more grand mal episodes without recovering from the first. This dog may actually be in a seizure for hours. This is termed "status epilepticus" and is usually referred to simply as "status." Seizures by themselves are not life-threatening unless they progress into status, in which case medical attention should be sought immediately.

Idiopathic Epilepsy

Idiopathic epilepsy, also called primary epilepsy, means that there is no identifiable brain abnormality other than seizures. Idiopathic, from the Greek language, is a combination of "idio," meaning "one's own or personal," and "pathy," meaning "disease." So idiopathic means "one's own disease." Studies report that idiopathic epilepsy (the single most common canine seizure disorder) occurs in 0.5 to 5.7 percent of all dogs. Most dogs with idiopathic epilepsy suffer their first seizure between the ages of one and five years of age. A genetic basis for idiopathic epilepsy is strongly suspected in several breeds, including the beagle, Belgian tervuren, keeshond, dachshund, British alsatian, Labrador retriever, golden retriever and collie. Idiopathic canine epilepsy may have an inherited basis in other breeds also.

Status Epilepticus

Status epilepticus is a serious and life-threatening situation. It is characterized by a seizure that lasts more than five minutes or a very brief break in between. Unless intravenous anticonvulsants are given immediately to stop the seizure activity, the dog may die or suffer irreversible brain damage. If status epilepticus occurs, you must seek treatment by a veterinarian immediately.

Structural Epilepsy (Symptomatic)

Structural epilepsy, or sometimes called symptomatic epilepsy, occurs when a tumor, infection, a head injury, or stroke affect the brain. These are seizures that are the consequence of an identifiable lesion or other specific cause. Dogs are less responsive with medication with this abnormality. With this type of epilepsy, surgery to repair tissue or remove a tumor is the best way for recovery. The extent and severity of damage and the outcome of the surgery will determine if seizures will be eliminated.

Reactive Seizures

Reactive seizures – Liver or kidney disease, low blood sugar, environmental toxins, or direct trauma are instances of reactive seizures. Any problem originating outside a perfectly normal brain are considered reactive seizures.

Cluster Seizures

Cluster seizures – More than one seizure occurs in twenty-four hours. Cluster seizures are usually caused by toxins or structural problems within the brain that continue to excite neurons even when they are exhausted and would normally be recuperating.

Partial Seizures (Focal Seizures) or Petite Mal

Partial seizures typically affect only a small part or one side of the body. These are often caused by a brain lesion. Partial seizures can be simple such as facial twitching or excessive pawing or biting of a body part. Partial seizures are also called focal seizures, and as the name indicates, the electrical storm is affecting only a part of the brain. A partial seizure may stay localized or it may expand to the whole brain and cause a tonic-clonic seizure. Because the seizure starts in only a part of the brain, an underlying disease or injury is highly suspected. A partial seizure may remain localized or spread to other parts of the cerebral cortex, producing a sequential involvement of other body parts.

They can also be more complex (psychomotor seizures) and cause bizarre behavior changes such as howling incessantly, biting at the air (fly biting), and aggression without provocation. Partial seizures are also called focal seizures, and as the name indicates, the electrical storm is affecting only a part of the brain. A partial seizure may stay localized, or it may expand to the whole brain and cause a tonic-clonic (Grand Mal) seizure. Because the seizure starts in only a part of the brain, an underlying disease or injury is highly suspected. A partial seizure may remain localized or spread to other parts of the cerebral cortex, producing a sequential involvement of other body parts. The dog is usually alert and aware of his surroundings.

Simple and Complex Partial Seizures

There are two main types of partial seizures: the simple partial seizure and the complex partial seizure. In the simple partial seizure, the dog will be conscious and aware of his surroundings, but confused. In the complex partial seizure, the dog is unaware of where he's at and displays abnormal behavior.

Simple Partial Seizure

In a simple partial seizure, the location in the brain that controls movement is affected, with the face being the primary place that is affected, with blinking and twitching on one side only. This seizure type may spread to the limbs on the same side of the body, with twitching and bucking. At this time the dog is usually alert and aware of his surroundings but is confused. The simple partial seizure may lead to a full-blown seizure (grand mal) or it may just stop and end the episode.

Complex Partial Seizure (Psychomotor Seizure)

A complex partial seizure will originate in the area of the brain that controls behavior or movement and is sometimes called a psychomotor seizure (see psychomotor seizure). During this type of seizure, a dog's consciousness is altered and he may exhibit bizarre behavior such as unprovoked aggression or extreme irrational fear. He may run uncontrollably, engage in senseless, repetitive behavior, or have fly snapping episodes where he appears to be biting at imaginary flies. The face is the area that is most commonly affected. Abnormal behavior, such as twitching or blinking, is observed usually on one side of the face. Thus, this type of seizure is asymmetric in nature. The dog is alert, aware of his surroundings, and confused by what is happening. This seizure might spread and affect other parts of the body as well. In such cases, buckling and twitching of the limbs might be observed. Examples of abnormal behavior are lip smacking, hysterical running, aggression, biting, hiding or crouching, and fly biting, when it appears as though the dog snaps at imaginary flies around his head. Such behavior is often accompanied by salivation, flank biting, vomiting, diarrhea, and unusual thirst or appetite.

Refractory Epilepsy

Refractory epilepsy occurs when anticonvulsant medications don't control the seizures. Usually these seizures are caused by structural problems within the brain, such as tumors. Thus, refractory epilepsy is usually a form of secondary epilepsy.

The Tonic-Clonic (Grand Mal) Seizure

The tonic-clonic seizure was formally called the grand mal seizure and is the most common of all dog seizures. The dog loses consciousness, falls to his side, and begins convulsing. The term used, tonic-clonic, is defined as the tonic phase where the body's muscles becomes rigid (tonic), and the clonic phase, in which the body's muscles has uncontrolled jerking (clonic). Often the dog will have facial twitching as his head is drawn back, and some involuntary vocalization. His eyes will be open, but the dog will not see anything. The dog will not be able to control his body functions, and will drool along with urinating and defecating. Once the tonic portion of the seizure is done, the dog will go into the clonic phase. Here the dog will go into rhythmic motion, like he is running or dog paddling, while chomping on an invisible bone. This will last a couple of minutes and then the dog will lie still for a while and then get up as if awaking from sleep. The dog may seem disoriented and begin to pace the floor and act groggy for some time.

A tonic-clonic seizure in dogs is one that affects the whole brain. This type of seizure is commonly seen in dogs with epilepsy, but can occur in dogs without this condition. Knowing the symptoms of a tonic-clonic seizure can help a pet owner know when a dog is about to or is having an episode.

Psychomotor Seizures (Complex Partial Seizure)

Psychomotor seizure is an older term used to describe a complex partial seizure, which is seen in its most common forms as either psychomotor or temporal lobe epilepsy. Psychomotor seizures are more complex than simple partial seizures because an alteration of awareness typically accompanies the experience of a seizure. A psychomotor seizure involves strange behavior that only lasts a couple of minutes. Your dog may suddenly start attacking an imaginary object or chasing his tail. It can be tricky to tell psychomotor seizures from odd behavior, but a dog that has them will always do the same thing every time he has a seizure.

Some psychomotor seizures are accompanied by a psychic stage. There are hallucinations, salivation, papillary dilatation, mastication, fecal and urinary excretion, and wild running. Seen in dogs with lesions in the pyriform lobe or hippocampus and from poisoning with agenized flour (canine hysteria). Called also running fits. The most common psychomotor seizure in dogs is the fly-biting seizure, in which the dog episodically snaps at imaginary flies. Seizures commonly begin with a pre-ictal phase, in which the dog may seem apprehensive or nervous, and they are frequently followed by a post-ictal phase in which the dog seems uncoordinated, confused, tired, and/or hungry and thirsty. Most seizures are between thirty seconds and two minutes in duration.

CHAPTER 4

When a Seizure Occurs

More than often the seizure will happen in the evening or at night when the dog is asleep, or in the early morning. Most canine epileptic seizures will occur while your dog is relaxed and at ease. It is very rare that a seizure will occur while he is exercising or at play. In addition, most dogs recover by the time you bring the dog to the veterinarian for examination. During the seizure, remain calm and clear the area around the dog so the trashing does not hurt the limbs of the seizing pet. Turn off any noise like radios, TVs, or music being played. Also shut off lights in the area because this will help with making a soothing mood for the dog coming out of a seizure. In a few dogs, seizures seem to be triggered by particular events, condition, or stress. It is common for a pattern to develop, which you will recognize as specific to your dog. Note that in some dogs a seizure trigger could be a certain event, like poison to their system, thunder, low blood sugar, or any other stressful condition. It may be you will never find the trigger because it is a physical anomaly like a brain tumor, which may require surgery. You will be able to recognize the conditions that cause a seizure by recognizing the common pattern (trigger) prior to the development of the event of a seizure. Was there smoke in the room? Loud noises like music? Is it a toxin the dog encountered in the yard or a substance he ate or drank? Did you treat the lawn with a weed killer, or use insecticide recently? By investigating and observation, you should recall if there is a possible trigger. There also may be a physical anomaly that would require a veterinarian visit to diagnose. As a seizure happens, the dog's body temperature rises, and he will pant heavily. This rise in temperature can damage the brain. Cool down the dog with damp cool towels or run a fan on low to lower the temperature. Most seizures are not life-threatening, but the seizure indicates a problem and you need to contact your veterinarian as soon as possible. If you think it's possible your dog was exposed to a toxin, you need to tell the vet. It could be something he ate or picked up in the yard.

Partial Seizures: Dogs can also have partial or localized seizures that only affect a limited part of their bodies. Formerly called petit mal seizures, these can be caused by tumors, abscesses, or other focal brain lesions. Owners of dogs with partial seizures may notice one or more signs of generalized seizures, but they will localize to a particular area of the dog's body. Dogs with partial seizures rarely lose consciousness, although they can have mental and/or behavioral changes.

CHAPTER 5

What Happens During a Seizure

During a seizure the brain is having abnormal electrical activity. This happens because of a number of disorders such as

- Abnormalities in the brain structure (possible head injury)
- Reaction to a toxin or allergen
- Reaction to medication
- Brain tumors
- Viral infections
- Bacterial infections
- Genetic
- Organ disease, liver, kidneys, etc.
- Idiopathic epilepsy (unknown reason)

Once the seizure starts, the dog is unconscious. They cannot hear or respond to you. Most dogs become stiff, fall onto their side, and make running movements with their legs. Sometimes they will cry out and may lose control of their bowels or bladder. Most seizures last between one and three minutes—it is worth making a log of the time the seizure starts and ends because it often seems that a seizure goes on for a lot longer than it really does. Dogs with seizures can have a wide range of involuntary, abnormally increased or decreased muscle activity. Generalized seizures usually start and stop abruptly. The actual event can last from seconds to minutes and is characterized by one or more of the following:

- Weakness
- Loss of awareness of the immediate environment
- Trembling
- Rigid extension of the extremities
- Cessation of breathing (for five to thirty seconds)
- Rhythmic jerking of legs while lying down (paddling; resembles running)
- Muscle twitching (especially facial muscles)
- Teeth chomping; chewing
- Frenzied barking
- Biting/snapping at invisible objects
- Temporary blindness
- Vomiting (emesis)
- Drooling (ptyalism)
- Inappropriate urination/defecation
- Collapse

Keep in mind that a dog cannot swallow their tongue during a seizure, so do not put your fingers on or near the mouth because you risk being bitten. While we cannot ask dogs how their seizures affect them, we can make reasonable assumptions by extrapolating from what people with seizure disorders tell us. Loss of consciousness, confusion, and trouble seeing. From what people with seizures tell us, dogs will not remember a thing about the seizure itself.

If the seizure lasts more than five minutes, or the dog has a cluster of seizures (multiple seizures in a twenty-four-hour period), the pet needs to go to an animal clinic or hospital for treatment.

Chapter 6

What to Do When Your Dog Is Having a Seizure

The first thing you need to do is remain calm. Panicking will only make your dog more anxious. Your dog needs you to be a calming presence to assure him or her that they will be okay. If there is something nearby that could hurt your dog during the seizure, move it out of the way. And definitely stay away from your dog's mouth, as you could get unintentionally bitten. Your dog cannot choke on its tongue, so you don't need to worry about that. If the seizure continues for more than a couple of minutes, your dog will be at risk of overheating. Turn a fan on your dog and pour cold water on his paws to help him cool down. As soon as the seizure ends, make sure to call your veterinarian.

If your dog has a seizure that lasts more than five minutes or if he has several in a row while he's unconscious, take him to a vet as soon as possible. The longer a seizure goes on, the higher a dog's body temperature can rise, and he may have problems breathing. This can raise his risk of brain damage. Your vet may give your dog IV Valium to stop the seizure.

What to Do If You See a Dog Having a Seizure

1. Remain calm.
2. Keep yourself safe. Seizing dogs can bite without warning.
3. Do not pull the tongue. Dogs don't swallow their tongues.
4. Using a hind leg, pull the dog away from furniture and stairs.
5. Cover with a blanket to reduce the light, and turn down sources of sound.
6. If the seizure continues, put an ice pack on the spine at the back of the ribs.
7. For transport to the hospital, use a blanket like a hammock to keep the dog, and yourself, safe.
8. Stay away from the mouth.
9. First off, dogs having a seizure can unintentionally bite you. Second, they cannot swallow their tongue, although sometimes they catch their tongue between their teeth and cause minor injury to the tongue, so there's no reason to get near their head.
10. If the dog falls on a hard surface, place a pillow under its head to reduce the risk of head trauma.
11. Dogs generate lots of body heat when they have seizures. They should not be wrapped in blankets, even if they are shivering, because the trembling associated with seizures rarely is caused by low body temperature.
12. If a dog has bumped into a chair or another solid object, it's best to move the object rather than the dog.
13. If the dog is on a couch or human bed, lower the dog to the floor, if it can be done safely. This will avoid any injury from falls.
14. Remove children and other pets from the area.
15. Observe your dog closely. Call your veterinarian if the seizure lasts more than three minutes, or if your dog has one seizure right after another. Severe and long seizures are a medical emergency and can be fatal.

16. The most important thing you can do if you're worried your dog may be suffering from seizures is to talk to your vet and get their advice. This is a serious medical issue and needs to be treated as soon as possible if you want a healthy, happy dog.
17. Keep a log of the time and length of each episode.

Immediate Care

A seizure, especially the first one, is a stressful, scary event for the dog owner, and you will feel powerless to comfort your dog, but you must take charge. While seizing do not try to move the dog, unless he in a position where he may be hurt, like the top of the stairs, sharp objects, or near a pool's edge. Move items close to the dog away so the dog does not hurt himself. Move other pets and children out of the room and dim the lights. Shut off any sounds like the TV or radio making noise. The dog may urinate or defecate while in a seizure, so you should have some tissue or toilet paper close by. You can comfort the dog by talking softly and petting as long as you stay away from the mouth where the dog could bite you with his uncontrollable chomping. If it's a mild seizure, you're talking softly to your pet may bring him or her around without a worsening seizure.

At this point you should write down a note of the time and place where the seizure happened and what the dog was doing just before the seizure started. This information is what the veterinarian will ask you. The most important thing to do is stay calm and hold your dog down. The dog needs you, especially when he comes out of his ordeal.

After the seizure, call your veterinarian and relay what transpired with your dog. If your vet is not available, contact the closest animal hospital or clinic. If the seizure lasted more than four minutes, take your dog to the emergency clinic or veterinarian immediately.

What Caregivers Need to Know

Yourself and people working with your pet need to be fully informed about the seizure diagnosis. They should know how to handle a seizure if it occurs, how to administer medication, and when to seek emergency care. They should also make sure the dog is eating and drinking properly to avoid dehydration, especially in hot weather. If a dog walker or trainer is taking your dog out, have her avoid excessive stress by taking the dog on walks individually (not with other dogs) and avoiding noisy streets and construction areas. Once the seizure is over, your dog may act as if nothing happened. But most post-seizure dogs will display altered behavioral characteristics for eighteen to twenty-four hours afterward. This includes confusion and disorientation as well as aimless wandering, compulsive behavior, momentary blindness, pacing, increased thirst, and even an increased appetite. Recovery may be immediate or take up to twenty-four hours. As a general rule, younger dogs seem to have more severe epilepsy. When the onset is before the age of two, the condition will respond positively to medication. But the more seizures a dog has, the more likely there is to be damage among the neurons in the brain.

Keep the Dog Cool

Dogs can overheat if they have a long seizure, so put cold water on their paws and turn on a fan to lower their temperature.

Prevention

Most forms of prevention will depend upon the frequency and underlying cause of the seizures. Your veterinarian may prescribe medication(s) or, if there is a behavioral cause (loud surroundings, etc.) to the seizures, the vet may teach you techniques for avoiding such triggers or direct you to a behavioral specialist.

Dietary management may also be recommended for small-breed puppies suffering from seizures due to hypoglycemia. These meals will typically consist of food that is high in protein, fat, and complex carbohydrates.

Most pet owners probably don't know this, but dogs can have seizures just like humans. Few things are worse than seeing your four-legged friend suddenly flop to the ground and tread water that is not even there, but for some dogs, this is their reality.

So how do you know if your dog has or may get seizures? And what should you do if they start experiencing them?

Stay Out of the Pool

Dogs suffering from epileptic seizures can drown while swimming if they have an episode, so it's best to find safer ways to play and exercise.

Nothing is more frightening and fearful as seeing your dog go into a full seizure. Your dog may be playing with a ball with you or just relaxing, then you look over and he's running frantically, flopping on his side with legs flaying, eyes glazed, teeth chattering, muscles twitching, and losing bladder control. This is the result of abnormal brain activity that can be caused by many different and varied problems. Some can be eliminated and some not. If there is a problem within the brain, the cause and condition is called epilepsy.

Epilepsy in dogs is the most common long-term neurological disorder with diagnosis and treatments that are straightforward with the veterinarian. The problem is that the decision to put your dog on seizure medication can be premature. The diagnostic tests can be negative, and a single seizure may be brought on by an environmental condition rather than epileptic or from a brain condition. If a vet says to wait and see what happens before a treatment, that may be increasing the harm to the pet down the road. There are many causes to a seizure, as you can see from this book, including environmental, toxins, tumors, parasites, medication, foods, medical conditions such as head trauma, and others. A comprehensive and detailed examination and testing need to be done to eliminate any possibility before considering epilepsy. Any epilepsy treatment to control seizures with medication can and will cause side effects, including adversely affecting the liver and kidneys, which, in itself, will cause seizures.

A Full Workup

A History

The dog with a seizure will need a complete workup, including a history of its health. What vaccine shots were given and when.

A Blood Count (CBC)

A blood count is needed to show what the white blood cells (for immunity) and red blood cells (for oxygen) along with platelets condition and count.

A Blood Chemistry Test

A blood chemistry test will indicate any reduction or increase in chemicals in the blood such as glucose (sugar) proteins, cholesterol, electrolytes, digestive enzymes, endocrine levels, triglycerides, aspartate aminotransferase (for liver function), and thyroxine (for thyroid function). Also included is a blood urea nitrogen (BUN) test, the creatinine test (CREA), phosphorus test (PHOS), and calcium test (CA) all for kidney function. The test for liver function is represented by six measured values. A test for Alanine aminotransferase (ALT), Alkaline phosphatase (ALKP), Gamma glutamyl transferase (GGT), Albumin (ALB), Total bilirubin (TBIL), and bile acids.

A Urinalysis Test

A urinalysis test can report the health of the kidneys and urinary tract as well as other organs. A urine test will measure the pH (acidity) and the chemical composition. High PH is associated with disease. Chemical analysis consists of protein in urine, glucose, ketones, blood, urobilinogen, bilirubin, and urine sediment. The last one is what is left in a sample after the test tube is spun in a centrifuge. The most common is blood cells, crystals, bacteria, and tissue cells from the urinary tract.

An X-ray

An X-ray can be used to see what is in the intestines as an obstruction, or any abnormality in the dog's skeletal structure.

A Magnetic Resonance Imaging (MRI) Scan

An MRI scan is used to scan the body or brain for tumors and anomalies. Not used much because of the cost; about $2,000 per diagnosis.

An Ultrasound

An ultrasound uses sound waves to see the dog's organs and blood flow from different angles in real time.

A CT Scan

A CT (Computer Tomography) scan is a computer-enhanced X-ray procedure to show detailed slices of images taken at intervals through the body or head. Like an MRI, this can be costly.

A DNA Test

The DNA test will determine if your dog has any genetic markers that are predisposed for diseases for that breed such as glaucoma, degenerative myelopathy, and dilated cardiomyopathy. This can also tell you your dog's exact breed or mix.

A Fecal Exam

This test is a microscopic examination of fecal matter to determine if any parasites are in the dog such as tapeworms or whipworms. Also if there is a bacterial infection, a fecal matter test will detect it.

Other Tests

Based on clinical symptoms, other tests include an electrocardiogram (EKG), cytology tests, ophthalmic tests (eyes), and biopsies.

CHAPTER 7

Care After a Seizure

1. **First thing, don't delay see the vet for a thorough workup.**
2. **Get your pet tested.**
   Your dog will need to have a thorough physical exam with a complete battery of tests. This will include a blood count, with a blood chemistry profile, a urinalysis, to find out the level of electrolytes, and a bile acid test to possibly find diseases especially in the liver. Tests such as an EEG, MRI, or CAT scan can determine if the brain is functioning correctly or a tumor is involved.
3. **Find the perfect remedy.**
   The remedies for seizures are as varied and numerous, but if the cause is truly epilepsy, then there is not a cure. But if it's caused by an unknown agent, biological, or physical, and can be treated, there are many remedies. Most all are addressed in this book from natural treatments, to medications, to diets, or homeopathic.
4. **Seek alternative methods.**
   There are many conventional treatments to seizures such as potassium bromide, Diazepam, Phenobarbital, and Keppra, but most of them have side effects that are worse than the cure. The alternative treatment with a more natural approach can be very effective in reducing the frequency

and severity of a seizure. Work with an alternate medicine or homeopathic veterinarian to find the best alternative treatment for your dog.

5. **Keep calm.**

   Your actions and how you appear after a seizure will be noticed by your dog. Try to remain calm, make sure your dog is comfortable, and be gentle to your dog. Your dog will be coming out of a confused state, start to pace, and be disoriented. Bringing your dog to the veterinarian after its first seizure. Seek immediate emergency care if your dog has a seizure that lasts longer than ten minutes or has three or more seizures in a twenty-four-hour period. She also suggests protecting your pets during a seizure so they're not in danger (i.e., falling down stairs) but do not handle them any more than necessary. They are unaware and can bite their owners.

Normally it is safe to approach a dog that is seizing—that is, unless you live in an area where rabies is prevalent and you are unsure if the animal has been vaccinated. Other important tips:

- Stay calm.
- Remember: the dog needs your attention, affection, and aid.
- At this time write down in a notebook what the dog was doing prior to the seizure, include the date, time, noise, odors, and weather. This will be useful information for the vet.
- Keep your hands away from the dog's mouth to avoid an injury. Although during a seizure a dog sometimes chokes on his tongue, this happens often with breeds with flat faces like Boston terriers and pugs.
- If this is a mild seizure, soothe the dog by talking softly to him to get the dog to relax.
- Get a blanket or towel and wait about a minute. If the seizure continues, wrap the dog in the blanket or surround him with cushions to protect him.

- When the seizure stops, unwrap the dog. This helps to prevent him from going into *hyperthermia*.
- If the seizure stops within four minutes, dim the lights (or pull the curtains) and make the room as silent as possible. In addition, keep other animals away and speak soothingly to the dog.
- If the seizure goes on for more than four minutes, take the dog to the vet immediately. Do not wrap him tightly in a blanket during the journey, as this may lead to hyperthermia.

After a dog has a seizure episode, your veterinarian will begin by taking a thorough history, concentrating on possible exposure to poisonous or hallucinogenic substances or any history of head trauma. The veterinarian will also perform a physical examination, blood and urine tests, and sometimes an electrocardiogram (ECG). These tests rule out disorders of the liver, kidneys, heart, electrolytes, and blood sugar levels. A heartworm test is performed if your dog is not taking heartworm preventative monthly.

If these tests are normal and there is no exposure to poison or recent trauma, further diagnostics may be recommended, depending on the severity and frequency of the seizures. Occasional seizures (less frequent than once a month) are of less concern, unless they become more frequent or more severe. In this instance, a spinal fluid analysis may be performed. Depending on availability at a referral center or teaching hospital, specialized techniques such as a CT scan or MRI may also be performed to look directly at the structure of the brain.

After a seizure, you need to contact your veterinarian as soon as you can tell your vet exactly what happens, how long the seizure was, and what you saw during the seizure. But if the seizure is nonstop and the dog is *still* seizing, he is having a grand mal and you need to take the dog to an emergency animal clinic or hospital for immediate care. If after a thorough exam and testing, and no underlying cause is determined by the veterinarian, it may very well mean the dog suffers from idiopathic epilepsy and there is no known cure and it is possibly inherited. The veterinarian, in most cases, will probably prescribe an antiseizure medication like phenobarbital, potassium bromide, or Keppra to control the seizures. It is important to remember there are many natural, homeopathic, or holistic treatments out there to look at that are known to give relief for dogs with seizures. Among these alternate treatments are:

- Acupuncture
- Acupressure
- Aquapuncture
- Laser acupuncture
- Electroacupuncture
- Aromatherapy
- Chiropractic
- Nutraceuticals (vitamins and minerals)
- Western herbs
- Chinese herbs
- Magnet therapy
- Essential oils
- Gold beading

There are probably others I missed or yet to be found, but these are the ones with the most promise to decrease a chance of seizure and even remove them from the dog's life forever. Always keep notes to track seizures with dates, time, severity, and any peculiar event that happened prior to the seizure. Sometimes the time of the month has an effect on a dog, like a full moon. With this information, your vet and you can be ready for the next event and have a plan to neutralize the seizure with a drug or other treatments.

Post-Seizure Treatments

After the seizure, treat your dog to a tablespoon of ice cream to bring his sugar levels back to normal. A seizure takes a lot of energy from your dog so you need to replace the burned energy as soon as possible or a second seizure can occur because of the low blood sugar. After the ice cream, feed the dog a small meal to help stabilize the blood sugar levels and calm them down. Another small meal in an hour or so will help stabilize the blood sugar levels in your dog.

Chapter 8

Diagnoses for Dog Seizures

How Is Epilepsy Diagnosed?

First, a detailed history is needed. A physical and neurologic exams are performed by your veterinarian, a panel of laboratory tests are run, and sometimes a CT scan or MRI of the brain will be recommended. If the cause of the seizure cannot be identified, the condition is diagnosed as idiopathic or primary epilepsy. There is no test to diagnose epilepsy per se. Our tests simply rule out other causes of seizures.

What Type of Information Can the Owner Provide to Help the Veterinarian Make the Diagnosis?

It is helpful if you, the owner, can give your veterinarian answers to the following questions:

- What does your dog look like when he is having seizures?
- What is the duration of each seizure and how often do they occur?

- Are there signs that only appear on one side of your dog (is one side worse than the other)?
- Has your dog had a high fever?
- Has your dog been exposed to any toxins?
- Has your dog experienced any trauma recently or years ago?
- Is your dog current on vaccinations?
- Has your dog been recently boarded or with other dogs?
- Has your dog had any other signs of illness?
- Has your dog been running loose in the last several weeks?
- What and when does your dog eat?
- Has your dog had any behavior changes?
- Do the seizures occur in a pattern related to exercise, eating, sleeping, or certain activities?
- Does your dog show different signs right before or right after the seizures?

Now That the Seizure Is Over, Can We Find Out Why It Happened?

After a dog has a seizure episode, your veterinarian will begin by taking a thorough history, concentrating on possible exposure to poisonous or hallucinogenic substances or any history of head trauma. The veterinarian will also perform a physical examination, blood and urine tests, and sometimes an electrocardiogram (ECG). These tests rule out disorders of the liver, kidneys, heart, electrolytes, and blood sugar levels. A heartworm test is performed if your dog is not taking heartworm preventative monthly.

If these tests are normal and there is no exposure to poison or recent trauma, further diagnostics may be recommended, depending on the severity and frequency of the seizures. Occasional seizures (less frequent than once a month) are of less concern, unless they become more frequent or more severe. In this instance, a spinal fluid analysis may be performed. Depending on availability at a referral center or teaching hospital, specialized techniques such as a CT scan or MRI may also be performed to look directly at the structure of the brain.

Diagnosis

Because there are so many underlying causes of seizures, your veterinarian will perform a number of tests to help determine the cause of seizures. These test will include CT scans and MRI scans to look at possible head trauma, bacterial or viral infection, or tumor. Testing the blood includes a CBC, chemistry panel, liver function test, blood count, and liver and kidney function. As mentioned prior, what is very important to the veterinarian is what occurred or what the dog was doing prior to the seizure. What was the environment prior to the seizure? Your veterinarian will need to know the dog's complete history, including breed genetic background, injuries, diseases, food, living conditions, etc.

PART II

CAUSES OF SEIZURES

Introduction to Part II

The Causes of Seizures

The Environment

The environment may contain many toxins and poisons. First thing you want to do is look at the dog's environment, his home, yard, where he sleeps, his walk to the park. where your dog plays and exercises. Is there anything that would cause a seizure? Think about the lawn treatment done on yours or your neighbor's lawn or even the park. The pesticides, insecticides, or herbicides used can and will trigger a seizure. Cedar shavings around shrubs are harmful as well as certain toxic flowers and plants. Extreme temperatures, cold or hot, can trigger a seizure in dogs. Bees, wasps, toads are potential environmental hazards for a dog. Antifreeze on the floor as well as floor cleaners are toxic. Did you buy a new flea collar? Cigar smoke, perfume, scented candles, air fresheners, loud music, and cleaning products are some of the environmental causes. Look at all the possible causes listed in part II of this book and investigate your surroundings. If you find anything toxic, eliminate it from your dog's world. If you're not sure of the what it is—toad, berry, or pesticide—take a picture of item and look it up on the Internet to see if it's toxic. Leave no stone unturned. Moon cycles also may put your dog at higher risk of seizures during a full moon. Speak with your vet about giving your dog Valium during these times to prevent seizures.

Health Issues

Does your dog have any previous health issues? Is his breed genetically prone to seizures? Has he had any head injuries? It would be good at this point to take your dog to the vet and have the dog checked out for infections, tumors, or a disease that can be a source of seizures.

Finding a Cause

If through your investigations of your dog's surroundings you think you may have found a cause for a seizure, gather up your evidence and make an appointment with your veterinarian for a checkup. Get your dog checked out for any physical anomalies to make sure your dog is okay.

CHAPTER 9

Disease

Disease in dogs can develop to a point where the dog can seizure. There are many diseases affecting dogs, and here is a list of some of the diseases that affect a dog's health and lead to a seizure.

Infectious Diseases, Including:

Viral infection – Rabies, canine parvovirus, canine coronavirus, canine distemper, canine influenza, canine hepatitis, canine herpes virus, pseudorabies, and canine minute virus.

Bacterial infection – Bruceellosis, leptospirosis, Lyme disease, ehrichiosis, Rocky Mountain spotted fever, clostridium, and kennel cough.

Fungal infection – Blastomycosis, histoplasmosis, coccidioidomycosis, cryptococcosis, ringworm, sporotrichosis, aspergillosis, pythiosis, and mucormycosis.

Protozoal disease – Giardiasis, coccidiosis, leishmaniasis, babesiosis, neosporosis, and protothecosis.

Parasites (internal) – Trichinosis, echinococcus, gnathostomiasis, hookworm, tapeworm, and yoxocariasis.

Parasites (external) – Fleas, ticks, heartworm, mites, cheyletiellosis, chiggers, demodicosis, and scarcoptic mange.

Cancers – Hemangiosarcoma, osteosarcoma, histiocytoma, malignant histiocytosis, mastocytoma, lymphoma, fibrosarcoma, squamous cell carcinoma, perianal gland tumor, anal sac adenocarcinoma, melanomas, leukemias, plasmacytomas, prostrate cancer, mammary tumors, oral cancer, ocular tumors, nasal cancer, thyroid cancer, gastrointestinal cancer, kidney cancer, lung cancer, heart tumors, testicular tumors, ovarian cancers, uterine cancer, bladder cancer, liver cancer, canine transmissible venereal tumor, and brain tumor.

Gastrointestinal diseases – Megaesophagus, gastric dilation, volvulus, anal fistulae, exocrine pancreatic insufficiency, pancreatitis, inflammatory bowel disease, bilious vomiting syndrome, intussusceptions, lymphangiectasia, and hemorrhagic gastroenteritis.

Urinary and Reproductive System Diseases, Including:

Kidney diseases – Fanconi syndrome, renal failure, glomerulonephritis, familial renal disease, and Samoyed hereditary glomerulopathy.

Urinary bladder disease – Bladder stones, urinary tract infection, and urinary incontinence.

Reproductive diseases – Prostate disease, cryptorchidism, false pregnancy, pyometra, umbilical hernia, and inguinal hernia.

Eye diseases

Eyelid diseases – Ectropion, entropion, distichia, chalazion, and trichiasis.

Lens diseases – Cataracts, lens luxation, and nuclear sclerosis.

Retinal diseases – Progressive retinal atrophy, retinal dysplasia, sudden acquired retinal degeneration, and retinal detachment.

Corneal diseases – Corneal dystrophy, corneal cancer, Florida keratopathy, chronic superficial keratitis, collie eye anomaly, cherry eye, canine glaucoma, ocular melanosis, keratoconjunctivitis, Vogt-Koyanagi-Harada syndrome, conjunctivitis, eye proptosis, Horner's syndrome, optic neuritis, persistent pupillary membrane, uveitis, asteroid hyalosis, synchysis scintillans, iris cysts, imperforated lacrimal punctum, and exophthalmos.

Ear diseases – Ear infections, deafness, and fly strike dermatitis.

Skin diseases – Allergies (including food, flea, and atopic), follicular dysplasia, dermoid sinus, lick granuloma, pemphigus, sebaceous adenitis, dermal fragility syndrome, discoid lupus erythematosus, and juvenile cellulitis.

Endocrine diseases – Diabetes mellitus, thyroid diseases (including hyperthyroidism and hypothyroidism), hypoadrenocorticism (Addison's disease), Cushing's syndrome, diabetes insipidus, and acromegaly.

Nervous system diseases – Syringomyelia, epilepsy, cerebellar hypoplasia, polyneuropathy, canine cognitive dysfunction (Alzheimer's disease), Scotty Cramp, Cauda equina syndrome, coonhound paralysis, tick paralysis, Dancing Dobermann disease, granulomatous meningoencephalitis, facial nerve paralysis, laryngeal paraysis, white dog shaker syndrome, wobbler disease, and cerebellar abiotrophy.

Skeletal diseases – Osteoarthritis, hip dyspasia, elbow dysplasia, Legg-Calve Perthes syndrome, craniomandibular osteopathy, hypertrophic osteopathy, hypertrophic osteodystrophy, spondylosis, invertebral disk disease, congenital vertebral anomalies, and luxateing patella.

Muscular diseases – Osteochondritis dissecans, panosteitis, and masticatory muscle myositis.

Cardiovascular and Circulatory:

Heart diseases – Degenerative mitral valve disease, dilated cardiomyopathy, congestive heart failure, sick sinus syndrome, atria septal defect, chronic valvular disease, myocarditis, dog heartworm disease, patent ductus arteriosus, pulmonary hypertension, hypertropic cardiomyopathy, subvalular aortic stenosis, pulmonic stenosis, ventricular septal defect, tetralogy of fallot, heart valve dysplasia, and cor triatriatum.

Circulatory diseases – Blood platelet disorders include thrombocytosis, thrombocytopenia, Von Willebrand disease, and hemolytic anemia.

CHAPTER 10

Chemicals

If you believe your dog has ingested a chemical substance that is poisonous to dogs, call a poison control hotline such as the one offered by the ASPCA right away (888) 426-4435 ($65 charge) or the Animal Poison Control Center (800) 548-2423. If you have the package for the product, check the label for   instructions. Do not induce vomiting unless suggested by a veterinary or hotline professional. Act fast to avoid causing permanent harm. If you see your dog suffering from seizures, is fading or losing consciousness, or is having breathing difficulties, bring your dog directly to an emergency veterinary clinic. Chemical poisoning can be lethal, so always act on the side of caution and call a veterinarian immediately.

Most common chemicals that are toxic poisons are:

Antifreeze (ethylene glycol) – One of the most common chemical toxic poisoning. Dogs are attracted to the sweet smell and taste. A tablespoon can kill.

Treatment includes inducing vomiting to empty the stomach and giving the dog charcoal to absorb the antifreeze in the stomach. A vet can administer medication that will prevent the antifreeze from damaging the liver and kidneys. Dialysis can be used to clean the blood of toxins and give the kidneys time to repair itself. If the dog is treated within twelve hours, the prognosis is good, but after twenty-four hours, the prognosis is grave. Symptoms are seizures, staggering, depression, increased water consumption, increased urination, and vomiting.

Cleaning products – There are literally thousands of household products on the market that can and will poison your dog and cause a seizure. Listed below are just a few of the cleaning products that are toxic to dogs.

Dishwashing detergent – Dishwashing detergent like Dawn are very harsh on a dog's skin and will make it dry and irritating to the dog. Stick with dog shampoo because it's made for dogs and is gentle on their body.

Drain cleaner – Common drain cleaners like Draino give off toxic fumes that are extremely harmful to your dog and make them sick. Keep your dog away from the room when applying drain cleaner.

Laundry detergent – Some laundry detergent is very toxic to your dog because they contain chemicals. Your dog may chew on bedding where detergent is not rinsed out.

Bleach – A dog will not try to ingest bleach because of the noxious smell that bleach has, but if you use it to clean your floor and your dog walks over the floor, the dog will stop somewhere and lick the paws to clean them and ingest the bleach. The dog will convulse, vomit, have seizures, and die.

Mothballs – Mothballs that contain the chemicals naphthalene or paradichlorobenzene are dangerous to dogs. Symptoms associated with ingesting mothballs with naphthalene include vomiting, diarrhea, anemia, weakness, and collapse. Symptoms of paradichlorobenzene include liver damage, staggering, or seizures. Call your veterinarian and read the ingredients to him or her from the mothball box. Your veterinarian will induce vomiting or administer activated charcoal or intravenous fluids.

Oven cleaner – Many oven cleaners contain ammonia as a degreaser. Ammonia has a very high-volatile organic compound that burns the mucus membranes

Pine-Sol – When cleaning floors with Pine-Sol or other strong floor cleaners, be sure it is completely dry before your dog walks on it and transfers the solution on to their paws.

Toilet bowl cleaner – If you have a dog who likes to drink from the toilet, they could ingest chlorine and other harmful chemicals found in toilet bowl cleaners. Always put the lid down and look for safe nontoxic toilet bowl cleaner that is available on the market.

Chemicals that cause seizures or convulsions: absinthe, acetanilide, acetone cyanohydrin, acetonitrile, acetylsalicylic acid, aconite, acridium Cl, acrylonitrile, aldrin, amanita pantherona, 2-aminopyrine, amphetamine, apomorphine, arecoline, arsenic trioxide, arsine, aspidium, astropine, barium, bromates, butacaine, caffeine, camphor, carbon dioxide, castor beans, cedar oil, chenopodium oil, chloramine T, chlordane, chlorinated camphene, chloronaphthalene, chlorpromazine, choke cherry, cocaine, coniine, corticotrophin, cortisone, cresol, creosote, cyanide, cyclotrimethylene, DDT, DFP, digitalis, dimenhydrinate, dimercaprol, dinitrobenzene, dinitrocresol, dinitrophenol, diphenhydramine, disulfiram, dulcamara, endrin, ephedrine, ergot, ethylene glycol, eucalyptus oil, fluorides, galerina venerata, gasoline, gloriosa superba, gymnothorax flavimarginatus, helvella, heroin, hexachlorophene, hydrogen sulfide, insulin, isoniazid, kerosene, ketamine, lead, beline, meperidine, mercaptan, murcury, metaldehyde, methapyrilene HCl, methyl bromide, methyl chloride, methyl formate, methyl salicylate, monochloroacetic acid, morphine, naphthol, narcissus bulb, neostigmine, nicotine, nitrogen oxide, oenauthe rocata, oxygen (100 percent, 3 atm), pantopon, parathion, phencyclidene, phenol, phosphorus, physostigmine, picrotoxin, pilocarpine, procaine, pyridamine maleate, pyrimidine, quinine, resorcinol, rhodotypos (berries), rosemary oil, saffron, sage (oil of), salicylates, santonin, senecio canicida, sodium fluoroacetate, squill, treptomycin, strychnine, tanacetum vulgare, taxus baccata, tetracaine, tetrachloroethane, tetraethyl pyrophosphate, tetraodontia, thallium, thiocyanates, thuja, trinitrotoluene, tripelennamine HCl, veratrum, Vitamin D, water hemlock, zinc, and cyanide.

CHAPTER 11

Medical Conditions

Health issues that can lead to dogs suffering seizures include liver disease, kidney disease, anemia, encephalitis, strokes, brain cancer, blood pressure that is too high (or too low), and electrolyte problems. Listed below are some of the medical conditions that can cause seizures in dogs.

Anemia (blood loss) – In adult dogs the most common causes of blood loss are trauma, slow gastrointestinal bleeding associated with stomach and duodenal ulcers, parasites, and tumors in the gastrointestinal tract. Symptoms include depression, weakness, breathing difficulty, jaundice, vomiting, hypothermia, and swelling of the face.

Bacterial infection – Leptospirosis is an infection of bacterial spirochetes, which dogs acquire when subspecies of the *Leptospira interrogans* penetrate the skin and spread through the body by way of the bloodstream. Leptospires spread throughout the entire body, reproducing in the liver, kidneys, central nervous system, eyes, and reproductive system. Symptoms include a sudden fever and illness, sore muscles, stiffness in muscles, legs, stiff gait, shivering, weakness, depression, lack of appetite, increased thirst and urination, rapid dehydration, vomiting, diarrhea, dark red speckled gums, spontaneous cough, difficulty breathing, irregular breathing, and runny nose.

Blood Parasitic Infections

Haemobartonellosis – Blood parasites are organisms that take up residence in your dog and are usually transmitted through the bite of a flea, tick, mite, or fly. The parasitic blood infection, haemobartonellosis, is a parasitic blood infection transmitted to our dogs by ticks and fleas. The red blood cells are targeted, and these are the cells that carry the oxygen in the bloodstream. They are highly antibiotic resistant, and are difficult to effectively eliminate. Symptoms are lack of appetite, listlessness, and whitish or purple gums. Babesiosis is a blood parasite caused by the protozoal (single-celled) parasites of the genus Babesia. Infection in a dog may occur by tick. Dogs that spend a lot of time outdoors, especially in wooded areas, are at an increased risk for tick bites and for contracting this parasite. Symptoms are loss of appetite, depression, weak, pale gums, and a fever. Dogs with an acute form of this disease can die from severe hepatitis.

Brain tumor (brain cancer) – Breeds with "smooshed" faces such as Boxers, Boston terriers, and pit bull terriers are overrepresented with brain tumors. Surgery may resolve seizures by removing brain tumors such as meningiomas, which are common in older dogs. CT scans can diagnose them early, but X-rays will not detect them. Older dogs tend to develop seizures from brain tumors. Symptoms are aggression, altered behavior, loss of vision, hearing loss, blindness, inability to walk, walking in circles, panting, and seizures.

Cancer – Cancer is the leading cause of death in dogs over the age of ten. But half of all cancers are curable if caught early. Symptoms are similar to humans, a lump or bump, a wound that won't heal, enlarged lymph gland, or abnormal bleeding. Golden retrievers have a strong incidence of cancer. So do boxers, flat-coated retrievers, and Bernese Mountain dogs.

Canine diabetes – Blood glucose levels that are too high (hyperglycemia) or too low (hypoglycemia). Low blood sugar can also be a cause. Diabetic animals taking insulin can develop low blood sugar-based seizures, or animals with insulinomas (a pancreatic tumor) Low blood sugar can also be a cause. Diabetic animals taking insulin can develop low blood sugar-based seizures, or animals with insulinomas (a pancreatic tumor)

Congenital defects – Congenital malformation (birth defects) of the brain stem or spinal cord is also a common cause of seizures. The Cavalier King Charles Spaniel is a breed well-known to have a birth defect in the occipital bone leading to cerebellar herniation, a condition known as syringomyelia.

Distemper – Canine distemper virus is a highly contagious disease with no known cure caused by a virus that attacks the gastrointestinal, respiratory, and nervous systems in dogs. A large number of species are susceptible to this infection. Besides dogs, coyote, wolf, raccoon, fox, mink, ferrets, wolverine, otter, and many other wild animals. The disease is spread through contact with an infected dog by way of respiratory secretions like saliva, sneezing, mucus, or contact with an infected dog's urine or fecal matter. Areas like kennels, dog parks, boarding facilities, and urban environments are all high risk for contracting the disease. Symptoms are a runny nose, discharge from the eyes, high fever, coughing, lethargy, vomiting, and diarrhea. Later, as the disease develops, it attacks the nervous system, and the dog will have muscular twitching, head tilting, convulsions, salivating, seizures and or paralysis. Treatments available include antibiotics, intravenous fluids to prevent dehydration, and anticonsultants,

Canine distemper is fatal in over 50 percent of infections, and the best way to protect your dog is a vaccination.

Electrolyte deficiencies – Electrolytes are the positively or negatively charged ions that circulate free in your dog's blood and other body fluids. They are the charged halves of the various salts that are dissolved in your pet's blood stream. The important electrolytes are sodium (**Na+**), potassium (**K+**), calcium (**Ca2+**), magnesium (**Mg2+**), chloride (**Cl−**), phosphate (**HPO42−**), and CO_2. The proper balance of electrolytes in your dog's blood is regulated by its kidneys under the control of antidiuretic hormone (vasopressin, ADH,

AVP) released from its pituitary gland, aldosterone produced by its adrenal glands, and parathyroid hormone (**PTH**) produced by the parathyroid glands in its neck. The signs of electrolyte disturbances in dogs include changes in your dog's breathing, irregular heart rate, muscle weakness, anxiety, vomiting, diarrhea, and depression.

Encephalitis (brain infection) – Encephalitis is an inflammation of the brain. Symptoms include fever, depression, behavior and personality changes (especially aggression), uncoordinated gait, seizures, stupor, and coma. Canine distemper is the most common cause of encephalitis in dogs.

Fungal infections – Fungi are widely spread throughout the environment, and many types of fungi are spread via airborne spores, which can potentially gain entrance to the body through the respiratory tract or skin. Fungi may either involve the skin or mucous membranes, or in some cases become widespread and involve multiple organs, including the lungs, liver, and brain. While hygiene is important in managing and handling dogs with fungal infections, treatment involves the use of specific antifungal drugs. Many of these diseases can be effectively controlled, but a cure is often difficult. Here are five of the most common fungal diseases:

- **Aspergillosis** is an fungal infection caused by the aspergillus, a common mold that lives indoors and outdoors in dust, grass, dead leaves, and other decaying vegetation. The mold spores float in the air, and a dog can easily inhale them. Dogs usually prevent infection by trapping the spores in the nasal mucus and expelling them with a sneeze. Symptoms may include sneezing, chronic nasal discharge, nasal pain, inflamed nostrils, decreased appetite, vomiting, fever, and weight loss. Breeds with long noses are more susceptible to infection by mold spores.
- **Blastomycosis** is a yeastlike fungal disease caused by fungus inhaled from decayed rotted organic wood. The fungus is most prevalent in the eastern states and southern Canada. Dogs are more susceptible than any other species.

Symptoms include fever, weight loss, loss of appetite, and depression. Advanced cases involve lameness, infection of the eyes, coughing, and seizures.

- **Cryptococcosis** – Cryptococcosis is caused by a fungus, *Cryptococcus neoformans*, which is widespread in the environment and can infect dogs. Dogs contract the *Cryptococcus* infection primarily by inhaling the fungal particles. After the particles are inhaled, they can take up residence in the nasal cavities or lungs. Symptoms are loss of motor control, loss of vision, weight loss, loss of appetite, fever and nasal discharge.
- **Histoplasmosis (Ohio River Valley fever)** is a fungal infection of dogs carried on dust, and is inhaled by a dog to infect his lungs. Found in the Midwestern states in the United States, in places heavily contaminated by bat, chicken, and bird dropping. Symptoms are varied but include fever, depression, loss of appetite, weight loss, coughing, labored breathing, and diarrhea. If the disease becomes worse, the veterinarian could find an enlarged liver, skin lesions, ulcers in the intestinal tract, or throat and eye infections.
- **Coccidiomycosis (Valley Fever)** comes from inhaling fungal spores from dry dusty soil in the southwestern United States. The spores start out in the lungs and then spread to the rest of the dog's body through the blood system. The coccidiomycosis fungal infection is a deadly disease and the most severe and life-threatening of the systemic fungal diseases in dogs. After exposure to the fungus, it takes seven to ten days to show signs. Symptoms include fever, lethargy, difficult breathing, coughing, weight loss, lameness, ulcers on the skin, and inflammation of the eye.
- Treatment is with antifungal medication for six to twelve months. The most common medications are Ketoconazole, Fluconazole, and Itaconazole.

Hyperglycemia is a high level of blood sugar (glucose) in the blood. Dogs, like people, need glucose for a source of energy, but need to maintain a range of 75 to 120 mg. If the glucose is too high or too low, it's a result of production of insulin at the pancreas. Causes of high blood sugar are pancreatitis, or the inability of the dog's pancreas to supply insulin. Other causes are tumors, kidney infection, urinary tract infection, dental infection, stress, exertion, and reaction to medications. Symptoms include frequent urination, increased amounts of water, weight loss, dehydration, cataracts, bloodshot eyes, dry nose, and nonhealing wounds,

Hyperkalemia – Hyperkalemia is the condition of a high concentration of potassium in the blood. Another term for this condition is Addison's disease. The heart rate of a dog suffering from hyperkalemia may be slower than normal. The condition may show itself as a generalized weakness in the dog and the condition becomes worse with exercise.

Hyperlipoproteinemia – A defective lipid metabolism causes this disorder. Lipids are classified as simple and complex. Simple lipids do not contain fatty acids. Complex lipids are essentially fatty acids and include glycerides, glycolipids, phospholipids, and waxes (ear wax). Lipids can combine with proteins to form lipoproteins. Apparently this disorder does not properly break down the fatty acids in the blood and the affected dog may have seizures. The Miniature Schnauzer is the most commonly affected dog. A high concentration of lipids (triglycerides) in the blood is known as hyperlipemia. Other clinical signs of hyperlipemia include dullness, poor appetite, and rapid loss of body condition.

Hypocalcemea – This is an endocrine disorder (affects electrolyte, calcium, magnesium, and phosphorous) that is characterized by low levels of calcium. Typically the acceptable range of calcium levels from the blood serum chemistry is in the range of 8.5 to 11.0 (mg/dl). Loss of appetite in a dog will cause the calcium levels to decrease, which in turn may cause seizures. Some dogs may develop muscle weakness early in the disease. Another symptom of hypocalcemia is cataracts.

Hypoglycemia – A dog with hypoglycemia (low blood sugar) usually has seizures prior to feeding when their blood sugar or glucose levels are at a low level. The signs of hypoglycemia depend on (1) level of the blood glucose and (2) the rate the glucose level drops. Some of the causes of hypoglycemia are a pancreatic tumor that produces an insulin like substance, liver disease, cortisone deficiency, diabetic dogs that obtain an insulin overdose

Hypothroidism – Other metabolic conditions such as hypothyroidism can also cause seizures. Interestingly, in one study 70 percent of dogs that had clinical hypothyroid had a history of seizures. I strongly recommend all dogs that have seizures be tested for hypothyroidism. Interestingly, in one study 70 percent of dogs that were clinically hypothyroid had a history of seizures.

Hypoxia or hypoxemia – Hypoxia (hypoxemia) is a condition of low blood oxygen levels that results in reduction in the capability of the red blood cells to carry oxygen. It may be the result of a disease of the lungs that prevents an adequate supply of oxygen getting to the brain, thus causing seizures.

Intestinal parasitic infections – Most dogs develop intestinal parasites, commonly called worms, in their lifetime because of their nature and lifestyle, being outside in yards or a park where a dog can walk on other dogs' feces then lick his paw, ingesting eggs of the parasite or worm. Also poor kennel sanitary conditions Some of these parasites can be transferred to humans if a person handles soil that had been in contact with dog feces. Sometimes you will not know if your dog has an internal parasite because of a few outward signs when they are first infected, but as the parasites become numerous, there will be symptoms that show a parasitic infection. There may be vomiting or diarrhea, because of the location of the parasites in the digestive tract causing irritation, although if the dog has lungworm or heartworms, this symptom will not be present. Parasites often will be present in the stool. Loss of appetite and fatigue because the dog is not getting his proper nutrients. The dog will have dry skin and the coat will be coarse with a loss of hair. Coughing will occur only if the dog has heartworm or lungworm.

- **Hookworms** – The hookworm attaches itself to the intestinal wall with its teeth and sucks the dog's blood. Hookworms are very small and are not seen in the dog's stool or vomit. Dogs can get hookworms from soil that is contaminated by the hookworm larvae. Dogs with hookworms can have millions of eggs in its stool. Symptoms from hookworms are weakness, anemia, diarrhea, and or weight loss.

- **Roundworms** are the most common intestinal parasite in a dog and like most intestinal parasites, the larvae are ingested from contaminated soil, from dog feces. Once the adult worm is in the intestines, the eggs are shed in the stool to the ground where they become larvae and the cycle starts again. Symptoms are diarrhea, vomiting, weight loss, and a shabby coat.
- **Tapeworms** – A long flatworm is a parasite to a flea. If a dog bites at a flea and ingests it, it will be ingesting a tapeworm. The tapeworm then attaches to the small intestine and grows its segments. The segments, which are egg sacs, break off and are excreted in the stool, and the cycle repeats itself. The symptoms are diarrhea, large appetite, irritability, and worm segments in the stool. Note that tapeworms can be transferred to humans.
- **Giardia** is a single-celled parasite and a common intestinal parasite. It lives in your dog's intestine and is contracted by dirty water or other dogs' feces. The symptoms are diarrhea, weight loss, and death. Giardia can be transferred to humans.
- **Coccidia** is a small protozoan single-cell organism that is contracted usually by puppies from the feces of the mother in an unsanitary conditions in a kennel, puppy mills, shelters, or animal hospital. The symptom is diarrhea, sometimes with blood in it, and in severe cases the dog may vomit. A cure is a drug treatment that takes three weeks.
- **Strongyloides** – Also known as threadworm or pinworm, it is commonly found in the places of high humidity and can be transmitted to humans. They come into contact with dogs, usually puppies in puppy mills, over crowded kennels or shelters when the place is in a dirty, unsanitary condition.

The larvae penetrate the skin or enter the dog from ingestion from present dog's feces. The symptoms are diarrhea and weight loss. Treatment is a deworming medication.

- **Whipworms** – As with other parasites, whipworm is transmitted by other dogs' fecal matter, but the eggs of the whipworm can live in an environment for up to five years to infect a dog. This makes re-infection more likely to happen. Once ingested by a dog, they go into the large intestine and make their home there. Symptoms are bloody diarrhea, and severe infections can cause death. Treatment is available from your veterinarian, but the yard soil where the dog contracted the whipworm needs to be treated as well or re-infection will result.
- **Cryptosporidium** is a highly infectious protozoan parasite that usually infects puppies because of their weak immune system. It is caused by ingestion of the parasite from contaminated fecal matter, water or food. Symptoms are diarrhea and fever. The veterinarian can prescribe medication to clear this infection up.

Lissencephay – A rare neurological disease in dogs suspected to be from a genetic defect within the brain and shows up in the first year of a dog's life and has no known cause. This condition is most prevalent in certain breeds such as Irish setters, Samoyed, Lhasa Apso, and Wire-haired terriers. The symptoms are impaired motor skills, growling at imaginary objects, aggressive behavior, self-mutilation, confusion, uncoordination, hyperactivity, and seizures. .

Liver disease – Liver function in the body is very important to a healthy life for a dog, and liver dysfunction is one of the leading causes of death in dogs. The liver purifies the blood, converts nutrients, produces enzymes that aid in digestion, and removes toxins from the blood. Causes of liver disease include genetics, where some breeds are prone to developing liver afflictions. These are Cocker Spaniels, Yorkshire Terriers, Rottweilers, and Dobermans. Some medications containing acetaminophen that can damage the liver and liver problems are common in older dogs. Other causes are bacterial or viral infections, diabetes, untreated heartworm, fatty foods, or cancer. Symptoms of liver disease include loss of appetite, jaundice, excessive thirst, weight loss, dark urine, diarrhea, vomiting, loss of energy, drooling, an enlarged abdomen (from fluid), seizures, and coma. The treatment of liver disease is dependent on the severity of damage the liver has. A change in diet in important to reverse the damage and begin healing the liver, as well as nutrients, supplements, and medications. The last option is surgery if there are any tumors, cysts, or cancer involved.

To avoid liver damage, have your dog vaccinated and maintain a good diet. Be aware of the medications taken by your pet and the effects on the liver.

Lyme disease is a bacterial infection transmitted by ticks by a bite. It is one of the most common tick-transmitted disease for dogs. Ticks get Lyme disease from infected mice and other small critters it feeds on. Ticks are in fields, woods, marshes, and brush, and wait for a host to come by to drop on to. Within twenty-four hours it begins to feed, injecting bacteria into the bloodstream. Ticks tend to attach to thin skin like the stomach, face, and ears. Once they are attached, they glue themselves to the host with a saliva and start to bore. Lyme disease is prevalent in the northeastern United States and somewhat in the Midwestern states. It is important that when your dog comes in from outside and you live in an area known to have ticks, you need to look for ticks on your dog and remove them. It can take up to five months after the dog is infected before symptoms appear. The symptoms are lethargy, joint swelling, pain in the legs (lameness), loss of appetite, depression, and coughs. In rare cases aggressive behavior and seizures can happen. If a dog lives in an area where ticks are known to proliferate and is exhibiting signs of Lyme disease, a visit to the veterinarian is needed to get a blood and urine test for the dog. An antibiotic treatment will usually clear out the bacteria and the dog will improve.

Renal (kidney) disease – The kidney's job in the body is to filter the blood, maintain normal red blood cell count, process the toxic waste in the blood, and turn it into urine, and conserve and balance the body water, acids and salts. If any of these functions are disrupted or slowed, renal disease occurs. This happens over a period of years and usually to older dogs ten to fourteen years old.

Symptoms occur over an extended period of time and vary. They include blood in the urine, lethargy, vomiting, increased urination, bad breath, lack of appetite, weight loss, depression, being thirsty, diarrhea, or constipation. The following breeds are prone to chronic renal kidney failure.

- English cocker spaniel
- Bull terriers
- Samoyed
- German shepherds
- Cairn terriers

An aggressive treatment is needed to bring back kidney function. The treatment for chronic renal failure is dieresis, a flushing out of the kidneys with an intravenous solution of electrolytes including potassium called fluid therapy.

The prognosis for chronic renal failure is poor, depending on the stage of damage to the kidneys, but with treatment and if the dog responds, the dog can live as long as four years.

Rocky Mountain spotted fever (see Lyme's disease)

Strokes – There are two types of strokes your dog might have. Both types involve a disruption in the flow of blood to the brain. An ischemic stroke occurs when the blood flow to the brain is disrupted due to a blocked artery. A hemorrhagic stroke occurs when the blood flow to the brain is disrupted due to actual bleeding in the brain, caused by a burst blood vessel. Canine stroke symptoms are tilting of the head, walking in circles, turning the wrong way when called, loss of balance, lethargy, loss of bladder and bowel control, and blindness. A severe stroke in the dog would lead to collapse and seizure.

Toxoplamosis (toxo) − Toxo is a disease caused by a germ (protozan parasite called Toxoplasma gondii), and the most likely places of contact are cat feces, raw meat, and uncooked vegetables. Approximately half of the people in the US have the toxo parasite, but the disease is dormant. This parasite is similar to Giardia in that once a dog has Giardia, it is dormant and may flare up at any time to affect the dog. Toxo has many symptoms and included in these are muscle spasms and seizures (neurologic difficulties). The symptoms worsen and the patient may go into a coma if the disease is not treated properly. The two most common drugs used in the treatment of toxo are the combination of sulfadiazine and pyrimethamine. Depending on the dog's reaction to these drugs, other drugs may be substituted: clindamycin, dapsone, or doxycycline.

Viral infection − Viral infections in dogs are different from bacterial infections in that they are much more difficult to treat, as a virus is much smaller than a bacterium. Some of the more common viral infections that can affect dogs include distemper, canine hepatitis, kennel cough, rabies, and parvovirus.

- **Parvovirus** − The canine parvovirus infection in dogs is a highly contagious disease. There are two forms of the disease. The first and the most common form is infection through the intestines. Symptoms are vomiting, diarrhea, lack of appetite, and loss of weight. The second form of parvovirus infection is the cardiac form, which attacks the heart muscles of mostly young puppies. The virus is spread by an infected dog's feces when a health dog sniffs the stool left. The virus can live up to a year in the ground. Vaccination is important for puppies to prevent the disease.
- **Canine distemper** − Canine distemper is a highly contagious virus that affects the dog's respiratory system, the gastrointestinal tract, and the central nervous system, as well as the eyes. Dogs contract the disease from other

dogs that cough or direct contact with saliva or urine. The first symptoms are sneezing, coughing, lethargy, diarrhea, vomiting, and eye and nasal discharges. Dogs not vaccinated are at a high risk of death if infected with canine distemper.

- **Canine herpes** – Canine herpes, also known as fading puppy syndrome, is an infection affecting the reproductive organ of adult dogs. The infection is transmitted by air (coughing, sneezing) and direct contact by sexual activity between the infected and the uninfected. There are no symptoms in adult dogs. Symptoms in puppies include lethargy, lack of appetite, trouble breathing, stomach bloating, blindness, seizures, and sudden death. There is no cure or vaccine for canine herpes.
- **Hepatitis** – Hepatitis is an infection that causes inflammation of the liver. The disease is spread by infected dogs' saliva, feces, and nasal discharge. Symptoms included are increased thirst, increased urination, fever, coughing, vomiting, loss of appetite, runny nose and eyes, jaundice, enlarged abdomen, and seizures. A blood test from the vet would confirm the infection, and there is no specific treatment. Vaccines are available and recommended.

Chapter 12

The Thyroid

The thyroid gland is in the neck and is an essential gland in the body, producing a number of hormones, including T3 (liothyronine) and T4 (levothyroxine), both of which are required for normal metabolism in the body. This thyroid disease is common in medium-to large-sized dogs, with some being more predisposed than others. These breeds include <u>Doberman pinscher</u>, <u>Irish setter</u>, <u>golden retriever</u>, <u>Great Dane</u>, <u>Old English sheepdog</u>, <u>dachshund</u>, <u>miniature schnauzer</u>, <u>boxer</u>, <u>poodle</u>, and <u>cocker spaniel</u>. It is also more commonly diagnosed in middle-aged dogs between the ages of four to ten years. Neutered male dogs and spayed females are found to be at higher risk than intact dogs. A vet would have a hard time diagnosing a dog with a canine thyroid disease because the symptoms can be contradictory. The dog may have diarrhea or constipation, greasy skin or dry skin, and lethargy or aggression. The dog may also have loss of hair, flaky skin, weight gain, muscle loss, ear infections, and intolerance to cold. A veterinarian will have to do a blood test called a complete T4 panel, which tells the vet the level of hormones in the blood, and this will determine if your dog has a thyroid problem. If confirmed, your dog will have to take an oral medication for the rest of their life, a hormone called levothyroxine or L-thyroxine. The dosage depends on the dog's size and weight.

Hypothyroidism – Hypothyroidism is a clinical condition resulting from a lowered production and release of T4 and T3 thyroid hormones required for the body. The thyroid hormone has many functions, but one of the most important is regulating metabolism. One of the main symptoms of hypothyroidism is weight gain.

Hypothyroidism usually is not detected until later in the dog's life, but new research shows that 90 percent of hypothyroid cases are caused by a genetic *autoimmune disease* called thyroiditis, which produces antithyroid antibodies in the body and may begin to develop as early as puberty, though clinical signs won't appear for years.

Hypothyroidism occurs when a dog's thyroid gland does not produce enough hormones. The thyroid gland is located in the neck and produces a hormone called thyroxine that controls the dog's metabolism or the turning of food into energy. This disease affects all breeds, but found that the following breeds are genetically prone to the disease: cocker spaniel, Airedale terrier, dachshund, Doberman pinscher, boxer, golden retriever, and Irish setter, at ages four to ten years old. Spayed females and neutered males also have a high risk of hypothyroidism. Small toy dogs and miniature dogs are almost never affected by this disease.

Symptoms include lethargy, hair loss, weight gain, flaky skin, intolerance to cold, excessive shedding, slow heart rate, diarrhea, anemia, ear infections, high cholesterol, and seizures. A blood test by your veterinarian is used to verify if your dog has hypothyroidism. The most common test is the Baseline T3 and the Baseline T4, which test the levels of the T3 and T4 thyroid hormones in the blood. If the tests show a reduction of the level of hormones, a synthetic hormone called L-thyroxine is given to the dog in daily doses.

Hyperthyroidism – Hyperthyroidism is a condition in which too much thyroid hormone is produced and it increases your pet's metabolism. This more regularly affects older dogs and can be a slow progression. Hyperthyroidism is sometimes caused by cancer, which may cause other symptoms to appear as well. Symptoms include weight loss, elevated heart rate, increased urination, hyperactivity, increased irritability, and increased appetite. In rare cases, your dog may become weaker with a decreased appetite and energy level.

Thyroid testing should be considered in any dog with recurrent seizures. In 77 percent of dogs with seizure, thyroid dysfunction was the cause. Although the relationship between hypothyroidism and recurrent seizures is unclear, thyroid testing is relatively inexpensive and carries little risk to the patient.

In North America, the principal reason for pet euthanasia stems not from disease, but undesirable behavior. While this abnormal behavior in dogs can have a variety of causes, there is a strong argument that there is a link between thyroid dysfunction and aberrant behavior. Typical clinical signs include unprovoked aggression toward other animals and/or people, sudden onset of a seizure disorder in adulthood, disorientation, moodiness, erratic temperament, periods of hyperactivity, hypoattentiveness, depression, fearfulness and phobias, anxiety, submissiveness, passivity, compulsiveness, and irritability. After the episodes, a majority of the animals were noted to behave as if they were coming out of a trancelike state and were unaware of their previous behavior.

Chapter 13

Genetics

Breeds That Are More Susceptible to Seizures

Any breed of dog can have a seizure and the cause can come from many things in a dog's environment. But many breeds hand down a form of epilepsy by way of a mutated gene that comes from the family tree (familial) of the dog's parent or both parents.

Some researchers believe that the mutant or recessive gene is the result of overbreeding and the cause of seizures and epilepsy. Four percent of all dogs will develop epilepsy.

Genetic epilepsy in dogs generally starts at about six months to five years of age, and most likely to occur at two to three years. Breeds that are more prone to inherited epileptic seizures include Australian shepherd, beagle, Belgian Tervuren, border collie, cocker, collie, dachshund, German shepherd, golden retriever, keeshond, husky, Irish setter, Labrador retriever, malamute, poodle, Saint Bernard, Shetland, sheepdog, springer, and vizsla. Other breeds that are more prone to seizures include the Finnish spitz, Bernese mountain dog, Irish wolfhound, and English springer spaniel. It's also seen in mixed breeds.

Dogs at increased risk are:

- **Small dog breeds** – with the tendency to have malformed skulls or low blood sugar. Seizures occur in small dogs that have malformed skulls, malformed brains, or hypoglycemia (a condition that occurs when blood sugar is too low). Newborn and infant pets of small-breed dogs, especially Chihuahua and Yorkshire terrier, are prone to seizures because they have little body fat and no significant carbohydrate stores to metabolize when their blood sugar is low (hypoglycemia). These pets also have little stomachs, so they cannot eat enough in a single meal to sustain them for a very long time.
- **Large dog breeds** – with shepherd or retriever genetics
- **Herding dogs** – with the MDR1 gene. Herding dogs with multidrug resistant 1 (MDR1) gene may develop seizures when exposed to particular drugs, such as ivermectin. Veterinarians in these cases generally prescribe drugs given daily for a specified period of time or a combination of lower dose medication in an effort to reduce the risk of seizures or other adverse reactions. Dog breeds that may have the MDR1 gene include the Australian shepherd, border collie, collie, German shepherd, long-haired whippet, McNab, Old English sheepdog, Shetland sheepdog, and silken windhound. See your vet to learn more about which drugs cause seizures and have your dog tested for the MDR1 gene.
- **Brachycephalic breeds** – with short, flat noses (bulldogs, pugs). Dogs with short, flat noses (brachycephalic breeds— pug, Boston terrier, and English bulldog)— may choke on saliva in their throat and airway and have difficulty breathing, so the oxygen does not reach their brain. They also have difficulty keeping their throats open while sleeping or while recovering from anesthesia. This is what causes them to snore and to have sleep apnea. Many brachycephalic dogs also have tiny nostrils, so not much air can enter the nose. Together, these anatomical features predispose brachycephalic breeds to seizures caused by anoxia (absence of oxygen).

- **Bull terriers** have an inherited form of epilepsy that includes tail chasing, irrational fear, and unprovoked aggression.

Pay Attention to Genetics

Genetics are important. When you get a puppy, ask if the parents have any history of seizures.

Know Your Pet's Health and Health of Their Ancestors

Liver disease can cause seizures, so you want to make sure that illness is not in the bloodline. This is difficult if you obtain puppies from pet stores, but if you have a purebred dog, the breeder should have this information.

Seizures can occur in dogs of any age, sex, or breed. Primary epileptic seizures and seizures caused by toxins, metabolic disorders, or conformational abnormalities are the most common in young dogs.

Chapter 14

Mycotoxins

Mycotoxins – A mycotoxin is produced by organisms of the fungi kingdom, commonly known as molds. One mold species may produce many different mycotoxins, and the same mycotoxin may be produced by several species. A **mycotoxin** (from the Greek words μύκης (mykes, mukos) "fungus" and τοξικόν (toxikon) "poison") is a toxic secondary metabolite produced by organisms of the fungus kingdom and is capable of causing disease and death. Mycotoxicosis is a term used to denote poisoning by food products contaminated by fungi (i.e., moldy bread, cheese, English walnuts, or even a backyard compost). As well as being toxic to humans, fungi release various toxins, also called mycotoxins, that are toxic to dogs.

Dogs allowed to roam or get into the trash may ingest tremorgenic mycotoxins, which are neurotoxins that produce varying degrees of muscle tremors or seizures that can last for hours or days. Toxins ingested in low quantities can cause fine muscle tremors that may last for several hours or days. With larger exposures, the tremors can become severe, progress to seizures, and may result in death. Tremors in cases of nonlethal intoxication may last several days. Vomiting often precedes the earliest tremors, which may help limit the severity of illness.

Mycotoxins are poisonous substances produced by foods contaminated by molds and fungus usually in spoiled food but can come from mushrooms, walnuts, or garbage. Depending on the amount of toxins ingested, the symptoms can appear in two to three hours. Symptoms include lack of appetite, muscle tremors, weakness, increased heart rate, panting, vomiting, increased body temperature, dehydration, and seizures. A vet will do a complete exam and a number of tests (urinalysis and blood) to determine and verify that your dog does have symptoms from a mycotoxin. Once it is determined that your dog has been exposed to a mycotoxin, the veterinarian will induce vomiting to expel as much poison as possible or give your dog activated charcoal to absorb the poison in the stomach. Intravenous fluids will also be administered to prevent dehydration, and an antibiotic.

Most dogs recover within forty-eight hours; however, ataxia, a condition where a dog will have trouble walking normal can persist for a number of years.

Mold in homes – Homes are a source of mycotoxins, and people living or working in areas with mold increase their chances of adverse health effects. Molds grows in houses when a certain dampness is achieved. Some of the mycotoxins in the indoor environment are produced by <u>Alternaria</u>, <u>aspergillus</u> (multiple forms), <u>penicillium</u>, and <u>Stachybotrys</u>. Stachybotrys chartarum contains a higher number of mycotoxins than other molds grown in the indoor environment and has been associated with allergies and respiratory inflammation. The infestation of *S. chartarum* in buildings containing gypsum board as well as on ceiling tiles is very common and has recently become a more recognized problem. When gypsum board has been repeatedly introduced to moisture, *S. chartarum* grows readily on its cellulose surface. The moisture controls and ventilation within residential homes and other buildings is very important. The negative health effects of mycotoxins are a function of the <u>concentration</u>, the duration of exposure, and the subject's sensitivities. The concentrations experienced in a normal home, office, or school are often too low to trigger a health response in occupants.

Mushrooms – Although various wild mushrooms contain an assortment of poisons that are definitely fungal metabolites, causing noteworthy health problems for dogs, they are rather arbitrarily excluded from discussions of mycotoxicology.

The severity and type of symptom will ultimately depend on the amount and type of mycotoxin ingested. Some of the more common symptoms associated with mycotoxicosis include:

- Muscle tremors
- <u>Seizures</u>
- Panting
- Hyperactivity
- <u>Vomiting</u>
- Uncoordinated movements
- Weakness
- Increased heart rate
- Increased body temperature
- Dehydration
- Lack of appetite (<u>anorexia</u>)

1.1 **In dog food – There were outbreaks of dog food containing aflatoxin in North America in late 2005 and early 2006, and again in late 2011.**
1.2 Numerous natural occurrences of mycotoxins in medicinal plants and herbal medicines have been reported from various countries including Spain, China, Germany, India, Turkey, and the Middle East. In a 2015 analysis of plant-based dietary supplements, the highest mycotoxin concentrations were found in <u>milk thistle</u>-based supplements at up to 37 mg/kg. Mycotoxins greatly resist decomposition or being broken down in digestion, so they remain in the food chain in meat and dairy products. Even temperature treatments, such as cooking and freezing, do not destroy some mycotoxins.

Even though Diamond, Country Value, and Professional brand dog foods have been recalled for containing highly toxic aflatoxins, they have caused an estimated one hundred dog deaths. Mold can be present in dog food whether it's "natural" or contains artificial preservatives, and expensive or low-cost. Conditions in the warehouse can determine if the dog food gets toxic. Always keep your dog food in a dry place. Buy smaller bags instead of large bags that take months to use up, so the product is freshest. Check the dates on the dog food bag for freshness. Do not dump bags of dog food into a plastic container because mold and moisture can accumulate over time in plastic. Any dry food left over in the container from an older batch of food can contaminate the newer food placed in the container. Check your dog food often by smelling it. If it smells "bad" or not fresh, throw it out or return it to the store and get some fresh, new dog food. Check your dog food store, your vet, or the internet for recalled dog foods, and keep the phone number available of the emergency poison center or the veterinarian. Symptoms that a dog has been poisoned by eaten toxic dog food are lethargy, vomiting, running nose, diarrhea, high fever, muscle tremors, and seizures. These symptoms can last twenty-four to forty-eight hours and can be life-threatening. Two-thirds of dogs die after eating moldy food. In severe cases, a dog will have blood in the vomit and/or a bloody stool.

Since mycotoxin poisoning from dog food can be fatal, treatment from a vet must start immediately. The first thing that a veterinarian will do is try to eliminate as much of the poison as possible by induce vomiting or pumping the stomach to remove the moldy food, or give the dog activated charcoal to absorb mold in the stomach. Medication could be given to the dog to initiate bowel movement. A blood test will need to be done to check the liver for signs of aflatoxin toxicosis. The dog will most likely be kept in the animal hospital for a day or two and put on IV fluids and antibiotics.

CHAPTER 15

Diet, Nutrition, and Seizures

Nutritionally related health issues can also be the cause of seizures. This is something many people never consider. When a dog has an epileptic condition with seizures, it's important to make sure that the dog has an optimum diet with all the nutrients that the dog needs. Some medications deplete the vitamins and minerals normally in a dog, as well as the disease itself can stress the body and require a supplement of nutrients. One of the side effects of seizure medication is an increased appetite, which is unhealthy to a dog if not controlled. A deficiency in a dog's diet can cause a seizure, and in a case of a dog with epilepsy, aggravate and worsen the condition. Improvement of a dog's diet and increased nutrients can help control and reduce seizures in a dog. Consult your veterinarian on the best nutrimental foods for a good diet for your dog and also investigate through the internet on what are the best and freshest dog foods available. You also may choose to feed your dog fresh raw foods you fix yourself, commonly known as "BARF" or biologically approved raw food. BARF is the practice of feeding your dog uncooked meat, bones, and organs in a belief that the dog is keeping with a more natural feeding process akin to the dog's ancestral wolf. In addition to raw meat, the diet would also include vegetables, fruits, and legumes.

Avoid foods with preservatives such as **BHA** and **BHT**, and ingredients shown as artificial coloring and artificial flavoring. Other ingredients to avoid are corn, soy products, casein, gluten, and dairy products.

Food Allergies

Dog food allergies are a becoming a major concern with dog owners because along with the itching and scratching, the dog is highly distressed. This can cause a systemic inflammatory response that can increase the dog's chances to seizure. Allergies are the results of a protein present in a grain contained in your dog's food. Your dog's immune system is mostly in the gastrointestinal tract and it's here that the protein gets broken down to be absorbed into the body. If the immune cells called enterocytes cannot break down the protein into smaller proteins, the cells are returned to the intestines for more digestion. If a damaged or poor functioning enterocyte lets the whole protein into the body, the next line of defense in the gut is the lymphoid tissue (GALT), which prevents the immune system from responding to a foreign protein and an immune hypersensitivity is formed. This is the cause of food allergies, which show up as excessive itching and scratching, dry skin, skin infections, ear infections, excessive licking, vomiting, and diarrhea. To stop allergic reactions, you need to change the food causing the problem. A vet may suggest a hypoallergenic diet that will not trigger an immune response, such as lamb and rice.

Pet Food with Chemicals

The pet food you feed can contain synthetic chemicals, preservatives, emulsifiers, or other ingredients that can cause systemic inflammation and increase the chance of seizures. Because many commercial foods are woefully deficient in key nutrients, the long-term effect of feeding such foods makes the dog hypersensitive to its environment.

If your pet has been on the same diet for a while or eats highly processed food, it could be a potential cause for seizures. Many pet foods and "treats" use chemical additives and food coloring along with other food ingredients such as wheat flour or wheat gluten, where evidence has shown these to be possible key activators for seizures. Such lower-grade foods and treats are often major contributors and should be removed from the diet.

Low Blood Sugar

Low blood sugar can lead to seizures. Supplement your dog's diet with carbohydrates and sugars per your vet's recommendations.

Blood Factors

Elements in the blood directly influence the brain. Among the most significant are sodium, potassium, chloride, calcium, glucose, and blood pH. For example, Chihuahua puppies are inclined to develop seizures because their bodies don't have reserves to maintain normal blood sugar levels. Lactating mothers develop seizures because their blood calcium levels are depleted by nursing young. This is most common when the puppies are three–four weeks old and have ravenous appetites.

Proteins

Protein is important to provide energy for dogs. Dogs are omnivores, which mean they are meat eaters like their ancestor, the wolf. Eating cheap dog foods, high in grain or corn, and low in meat protein is why many dogs have shabby coats and low energy levels. Dogs need beef, lamb, fish, poultry, and dairy, and the protein it provides. A dog needs ten amino acids, which come from protein from their food diet. Watch for deceptive labels that use the term "crude protein" as an ingredient because it can be misleading. Crude protein on a label is actually a chemical analysis of the food showing the amount of nitrogen in the food as protein. While nitrogen can come from an animal, it can also come from grain or from animal carcasses. Choose a food with whole meat as the first ingredient, whether its chicken, beef, lamb, or fish.

Amino Acids

Amino acids are the basic building blocks of protein, and of the twenty amino acids, there are ten amino acids that cannot be synthesized by the dog's body in sufficient quantity and must be supplied by the dog's food. There are called essential amino acids. These amino acids are arginine, histidine, isoleucine, leucine, lysine, methionine, phenylalanine, threonine, tryptophan, and valine. When you are buying food for your dog, read the label and see if any of these essential amino acids are included. Remember that all dried or canned dog food is heated in the manufacturing process and that will destroy the protein. Dog food manufacturers add "crude protein" usually from grains or animal carcasses, an inexpensive way to add protein and is not enough for a dog's daily requirement of protein. Make sure there is real whole meat on the label before you buy it. On a dog food bag, there is a list of ingredients. The ingredients are listed by the quantity amount that is in the bag or can. So if the ingredient is turkey, that would be the largest quantity ingredient in the can, and the last item on the list would be the smallest quantity of ingredient in the bag or can. Dogs need amino acids for strong muscles and nerve system in the body. Dogs who do not receive enough amino acids are susceptible to enlarged thyroid, poor growth, weakness, increased heart rate, gastrointestinal problems, joint pain, and seizures.

Nonessential amino acids are produced by the body and do not come from food. An important nonessential amino acid is **taurine.** This inhibitor amino acid is instrumental in the prevention and / or reduction of seizures in dogs. It has the ability to reduce activity in the brain cells, since epileptic attacks are an overstimulation of brain cells. Taurine is released during a seizure to protect the brain from damage. It's important to note that taurine can only be produced by the body if it gets enough animal protein, and a deficiency in taurine can cause epileptic seizures. Taurine also helps regulate blood sugar levels in a dog. Consult your veterinarian on a supplement of taurine to be administered if your dog has had seizures. It could be that the seizures are a result of a taurine deficiency in the dog, resulting in epileptic attacks.

Enzymes

Enzymes are small protein molecules found in cells in dogs that are used to initiate speedy food digestion, strengthen the immune system, aid in nutrient absorption, stop coprophagia (habit of eating stool), toxic buildup in the body supports health teeth, promotes normal weight, and decrease the risk of degenerate diseases. If there is a lack of food enzymes in a dog's body, the pancreas will be burdened to produce more digestive enzymes and cause improper food digestion and the growth of unwanted bacteria in the gut. There are two main groups of enzymes: metabolic and digestive.

Metabolic enzymes

Metabolic enzymes are produced in the pancreas, cleanse toxins from the body, send nutrients to all the organs of the body, help produce energy, as well as remove dead cells, and are the major component in cell reproduction and repair in all parts of the body. There are two ways to ensure that your dog has enough metabolic enzymes in their body. One is to eat enzyme-rich foods such as raw honey, bee pollen, melons, and papaya. The other is to use enzyme supplements. It is important though to consult your veterinarian before you give your dog enzyme supplements to ensure that there is no reaction with other existing medications.

Digestive enzymes

Digestive enzymes break down and convert ingested substances (food) to provide the nutrients needed to sustain energy for the body. The digestive enzyme is produced in the pancreas and released in the small intestine to break down the food. High levels of digestive enzymes are found in uncooked food that is being eaten, but also the pancreas secretes the amount of digestive enzymes needed to help in the digestion. There are four enzymes that are used to break down the food:

- Cellulase – breaks down and decomposes fiber
- Amylase – breaks down and decomposes carbohydrates such as starches
- Lipase – breaks down fats into glycerol
- Protease – breaks down proteins into amino acids

Digestive enzymes not only absorb nutrients and aid in digestion, but they also improve the immune system, minimize the risk of developing disease, enhance cell production, and promote weight loss. If the dog lacks digestive enzymes and the pancreas cannot supply enough enzymes to properly digest food, the undigested carbohydrates, fats, and proteins promote the growth of bacteria that upset the balance in the gut and cause malnutrition. The results are bloating, gas, bad breath, diarrhea, body odor, weight loss, and lethargy. Along with this come compromised immune system, cancer, allergies, skin problems, and arthritis. A proper exam by your vet will determine if there's a lack of digestive enzymes. He will have to do a urinalysis, blood count, stool analysis, and a pancreatic function test to diagnose your pet. The majority of dogs will be successfully treated by over-the-counter or prescription supplement. Dogs low in enzymes are usually deficient in vitamins and minerals and will also need those supplements to stabilize their health.

Vitamins

Vitamins are an organic compound and are essential for normal growth and development in a body. They are nutrients absorbed from food intake and react in the body to produce skin, organs, bone, and muscle. Most nutrients are found in natural foods and are in most commercially processed dog food. Because vitamins are destroyed by heat in the manufacturing process, dogs may need to have a vitamin supplement to maintain a healthy level of nutrients required to protect the dog from disease and dysfunction caused by lack of vitamins. Also check the label on the food that the dog is eating. Some commercial dog foods contain added vitamins as an ingredient to their foods, but not enough to make a difference due to state regulations. A prescribed dog food will have a therapeutic dose of vitamins and contain enough supplements to maintain a level of health. There are various vitamin deficiencies that are specifically linked to seizures in dogs.

Vitamin A

Vitamin A, also called carotene, is a fat-soluble antioxidant vitamin that is stored in the liver. It is needed for a dog's skin, coat, vision, muscles, and more. Sources of vitamin A include dairy products, fish oil, liver, dark fruits and vegetables, and egg yolks. The problem with vitamin A is that since it is fat-soluble and stored in the liver, excess vitamin A cannot be excreted or eliminated from the body like water-soluble vitamins, which means it can reach high toxic levels within the dog's body. Toxicity occurs usually when an owner feed their dog, usually puppies, supplemental vitamin A or too much fish liver oil. Symptoms of canine toxicity are weight loss, stiffness, lethargy, no appetite, and weakness.

Vitamin B

Vitamin B is called B complex because it includes eight types. They are vitamin B1 (thiamine), vitamin B2 (riboflavin), vitamin B3 (niacin), vitamin B5 (pantothenic acid), vitamin B6 (pyridoxine), vitamin B7 (biotin), vitamin B9 (folic acid), and vitamin B12 (cobalamin). The vitamin B complex is a group of water-soluble vitamins found in unprocessed foods and added to some commercial dog foods as a supplement (check the label). Because vitamin B complex is water-soluble, excess vitamins are readily excreted out the body. Excellent sources of B vitamins are turkey, tuna, and liver. Also beans and whole grains. Deficiency of vitamin B is well-known as a cause for seizures in canines. Because commercial foods are cooked and destroy these vital vitamins, either a raw diet or vitamin supplements are required especially for seizure dogs. Deficiency in vitamin B6 has been known to cause seizures in dogs, but an excess of vitamin B6 can cause ataxia (loss of balance) and possibly liver disease.

Vitamin C

Vitamin C, also known as ascorbic acid, is essential nutrient found in numerous fruits and vegetables such as apples, green beans, and sweet potatoes. (Note: Do not give a dog a whole apple since the seeds in the core contain cyanide, which is a poison.) Dogs can produce vitamin C in their body from sunlight, but if a dog is sick or stressed, the dog can cause the depletion of vitamin C. Vitamin C is vital for dogs because it boosts the immune system, protects against numerous diseases, and gives the dog to recover from an injury or illness. It also acts as an anticarcinogen in dogs, protects against allergies, and helps in several bacterial or viral infections.

Vitamin D

Vitamin D is a fat-soluble vitamin like vitamin A that is stored in the liver and is vital for bone, nerve, and muscle health in your dog. It also regulates calcium in the kidneys and the body. High levels of vitamin D from drugs or diet can cause toxicity in dogs; usually puppies are at a higher risk. One cause of vitamin D toxicity in dogs is the ingestion of rat poison chemicals.

Vitamin E

Vitamin E is an essential and important antioxidant that plays a crucial role in your dog's health. Vitamin E protects cells and helps cells repair damage caused by free radicals, a group of atoms produced by the body or an outside source, usually a toxin or pollutant. Most commercial dog food has the minimum amount of vitamin E needed to maintain a healthy diet, and a deficiency is rare in dogs. Vitamin E can be found in green leafy vegetables and plant oils. Vitamin E deficiency is known to cause seizures, and adding vitamin E as a supplement to a diet can reduce seizure frequency in dogs afflicted with epilepsy.

Minerals

The presence of minerals in dogs is essential for health and plays an important part in a dog's nutrition. Minerals aid in the formation of bone, oxygen in the blood, and normal muscle and nerve function. Minerals are divided in to two groups. The high-quantity groups, known as macrominerals, are calcium, phosphorus, potassium, sodium, and magnesium. The low-quantity groups, known as microminerals (trace minerals), are selenium, manganese, zinc, copper, iron, chromium, and iodine. The macrominerals are required in greater amounts in a dog's body, while the microminerals are needed in smaller quantities. Deficiency in minerals dogs can cause anemia, dehydration, and lead to more serious health conditions. Mineral deficiency is known to cause or aggravate seizures in dogs. Most commercial dog food contains the minimum daily amount for dogs, but every dog is different in age, breed, size, metabolism, and activity level, which will require a higher need for additional minerals. For these dogs, a nutritional supplement should be considered. Always ask your veterinarian to assess your dog's needs and recommend a good supplement.

Magnesium

Magnesium is a key nutrient mineral involved with energy production at a cellular level to move muscles and transfer the energy where it's required as well as proper bone growth, and is needed for the absorption of certain other minerals and vitamins. It is the second most abundant mineral in the dog's body. Magnesium can be found in milk, fish, whole grains, soybeans, and wheat germ, although cooking can remove the mineral from the food. Magnesium is the second most abundant substance in cells, behind potassium, so a deficiency in magnesium is a serious health concern. In the body, 60 percent of magnesium is found in the bones and 40 percent is found in the liver and soft tissue. Magnesium deficiencies are rare and are mostly due to malnutrition. Its symptoms are muscle tremors, weakness, depression, incoordination, lethargy, and then seizures.

Manganese

Manganese occurs mostly in a dog's liver, but can be found in the kidneys, pancreas, and bone. It is needed for the proper use of protein and carbohydrate by the body and the maintenance of the nervous system. Manganese deficiency is rare in dogs, but if it occurs, it's usually in newborn or puppies, and its symptoms are ataxia (loss of equilibrium), poor growth, and eventually, seizures. Good sources of manganese are whole grains, eggs, nuts, and green vegetables.

Selenium

Selenium is an antioxidant that, in conjunction with vitamin E and enzymes, protects the cells in the body from cancer and aging, fights inflammation, and maintains thyroid hormone levels. Food sources of selenium are wheat germ, bran, brown rice, oats, tuna fish, liver, turnips, and barley. An important factor of concern is that in some farms, the soil many be deficient in selenium and vegetables grown in that soil will not have the mineral selenium in the vegetable. Selenium deficiency in dogs are rare, but is often prescribed as an antioxidant for dogs with epilepsy, inflammatory bowel disease, and cancer.

Calcium

Calcium is beneficial in dogs for bone growth, nails, teeth, and coat. Without calcium, a dog is more susceptible to osteoporosis, bone diseases, and heart problems.

Calcium can be found in milk, yogurt, cottage cheese, and cheese. Other sources are fish, salmon, tuna, sardines, and trout that are cooked, never raw. Do not feed your dog bones even though they are rich in calcium; a splinter can puncture an organ, resulting in death. Symptoms for a calcium deficiency are rickets, muscle twitching, lethargy, panting, stiffness, and seizures.

Zinc

Zinc is an essential mineral that is critical for canine body function, particularly the skin and coat. Besides supporting the immune system and improving energy, this nutrient is good for a dog's general health. Zinc is found in oysters and, to a far lesser degree, in most animal proteins, beans, nuts, almonds, whole grains, pumpkin seeds, and sunflower seeds, but studies show that up to 40 percent of zinc intake is not used by the body.

There is a fragile balance on how much zinc a dog needs to have. An excess of zinc and the dog will develop zinc toxicity. Symptoms include jaundice, depression, lethargy, diarrhea, vomiting, and lack of appetite. Causes are usually swallowing a toy from a board game, pennies, nails, staples, and some lotion. Too little zinc and the regeneration of hair, skin, and nails, and general healing are reduced. The best advice is to ask a veterinarian to test your dog's blood and see what the diagnoses is, and recommend a course of action, either a zinc supplement or a blood transfusion.

Diet and seizures

The main nutritional goal for a dog with seizures or epilepsy is to supply the nervous system and particularly the brain with as much rich nutrients as possible. This can reduce the medications that come with a harmful side effect, but can reduce the number of seizures for the dog.

A number of goals to consider for a good diet are:

1. Go grain-free. Grains have no nutrimental value for your dog. Wheat, soy, and corn are primary ingredients in low-quality dog foods. Besides not having any nutritional value, they are heavy with carbohydrates and calories instead of protein. Dogs have evolved as meat eaters from the wild and today's domestic dog is not that different.
2. See what's in your dog food. Learn to check the ingredients. Chemicals like **BHT** (a preservative), **BHA** (a preservative), ethoxyquin (a preservative associated with liver damage) and propylene glycol (found in antifreeze, used to keep dog food moist), along with artificial flavoring and coloring, are need to be avoided. Corn syrup is sugar and used to sweeten the food to make it desirable to your dog. It also causes diabetes and hyperactivity. You may even consider making your own dog food.

3. Use vitamin and mineral supplements to promote good health, especially for the brain. Most people rely on off-the-shelf dog food and this is okay, but the pet's diet may be lacking. Each dog has a different metabolism and has different needs. Check with your vet to find out what your dog is lacking through a blood test and diagnosis.

Chapter 16

Heatstroke

Heatstroke is too-frequent cause of seizures in pets and is a condition that results from hyperthermia (an elevation in body temperature). This increase typically occurs as a response to a trigger, such as inflammation in the body or a hot environment. When a dog is exposed to high temperatures, heatstroke or heat exhaustion can result. Heatstroke is a very serious condition that requires *immediate* medical attention. Once the signs of heatstroke are detected, there is precious little time before serious damage or even death can occur. Dogs do not sweat through their skin like humans. They release heat primarily by panting and they sweat through the foot pads and nose. If a dog cannot effectively expel heat, the internal body temperature begins to rise. Once the dog's temperature reaches 106°, damage to the body's cellular system and organs may become irreversible. Unfortunately, too many dogs succumb to heatstroke when it could have been avoided. Learn how to recognize the signs of heatstroke and prevent it from happening to your dog. Leaving a dog in a car on a hot day with windows closed, in the outdoors, or in a backyard without shade or water is just irresponsible and life-threatening.

Signs of Heatstroke in Dogs

The following signs may indicate heatstroke in a dog:
- Have trouble breathing or vigorous panting
- Elevated heart rate
- Dry and dark red gums
- Purple tongue
- Lying down and unwilling or unable to get up; listless
- Loss of consciousness
- Foaming at the mouth
- Dizziness or disorientation
- Seizures

The dogs with the highest risk of developing heatstroke are the very young and old, as well as long-haired dogs and brachycephalic breeds (pug, shih tzu, Pekinese, Boston terrier, King Charles spaniel, English bulldog, and French bulldog) due to their flat face, which causes breathing problems. A dog's temperature is normally between 99.5 and 102.5 degrees Fahrenheit. Take the dog's temperature with a rectal thermometer and if the temperature is over 103 degrees, the dog is in danger. It's fatal if a temperature reaches 109 or higher. Check the temperature every five minutes.

Immediate Care for heatstroke

Heatstroke can kill a dog in a short period of time, so the dog needs to be removed from the source of the heat, inside a car, or direct sun, to a shaded area or, better, an air conditioned area. Give the dog a bowl of water, but don't force the dog to drink. Take a clean cloth soaked in water and wet the dog's lips, gums, and tongue while squeezing the cloth. Place a cold cloth with ice cubes on the dog's head or even a frozen bag of vegetables from the refrigerator. If you're outdoors, use a hose to spray the dog with a light stream. If the dog is inside, place them into a tub and shower with cold water. Applying cold packs to the paw pads will help dissipate the heat. Applying isopropyl alcohol to the paw pads, groin area, arm pits, and flanks can enhance evaporative cooling also. Call your veterinarian, report the heatstroke, and wait for instructions. The dog will need to have a complete physical exam to assess if any damage was done to the organs or there's brain swelling, which could be fatal. The prognosis for dogs with heatstroke depends on how long the dog was exposed to the heat, but if the dog had a seizure due to the heatstroke, there may be other neurological damage.

Preventing Heatstroke

There are a number of ways to keep your dog from ever experiencing a heatstroke and possible death.

1. Keep your dog inside your house during hot weather, especially if you live in hot areas of the south and southwest. Watch for heat waves on the news channels and plan ahead.
2. Give your dog a haircut especially if they have a thick coat, but do not cut it too close to the skin because the fur helps keep the dog from getting a sunburn. But you want to keep your dog cool in the summer time.
3. Take your dog out to do their duty in the morning or evening hours when it is cooler. If the dog must go out in the afternoon, limit the time.
4. If you have to keep the dog outside during the day, provide shade, a tree, or dog house, and water. Two water bowls are better in case one is spilled. Provide a kiddie pool for the dog to splash around and cool themselves off. Check on the water supply and them often.
5. Never leave your dog in a car. The temperature in a car is always 30 degrees more than outside the car in minutes, and there is no breeze in the car. Dogs cannot cool themselves like

humans. They don't sweat, except for their paws. They cool down by panting.
6. Do not exercise with your dog on a very hot day. A regular routine will have to be altered if it's extremely hot outside. Go for the walks in the early morning or late evening when the temperatures are cooler.

CHAPTER 17

Vaccines

Few issues in veterinary medicine are as controversial as the debate about administering annual vaccinations to our dogs. Long considered part of the standard of baseline, responsible veterinary healthcare, and credited with conquering some of the fiercest canine viral and other infectious diseases, vaccinations now are also suspected of creating vulnerability to illnesses and chronic conditions such as anemia, arthritis, seizures, allergies, gastrointestinal and thyroid disorders, and cancer. Current debate in veterinary medicine concerning issues related to vaccine efficacy and safety as well as the duration of immunity induced by the currently available vaccines, underscores a compelling need for more objective and scientific data. Unfortunately, there is no accepted protocol for vaccinating dogs. Veterinarians have been divided with this controversial issue for quite some time, like the question of human vaccines.

There are two main camps on the subject of vaccinations of dogs.

1. **More Vaccines** - That dogs should be given vaccinations every year, with the logic that it's working with decreased cases of some diseases, why mess with it, and some bacterial vaccines like Lyme disease, bordetellosis, and leptospirosis are shown to be only good for a year and more so in some areas of high incidence of the contagions.

2. **Less Vaccines** - That vaccines should be given every three years because some dogs react poorly to a vaccination with immune-related disorders like anemia. There is no data to say how long a vaccination lasts in the body, but it's very likely over one year.

Should you vaccinate?

The question is do I vaccine my dog or not? Your dog needs to be vaccinated as a protection and defense against diseases. Not to vaccinate is to expose your dog to deadly diseases and spreading them to other dogs. The real question remains, do I vaccinate every year or every three years? I am on the side of every three years because of the side effects a dog is put through with too many vaccinations that are not necessary.

What is a vaccine?

A vaccine is an antigenic substance injected into the body to stimulate the immune system to develop immunity to that particular disease. Some diseases are too strong and can become deadly very quickly. A vaccine is part of a microbe that has been weakened or killed so that there is no threat to the body. The vaccine mildly simulates the immune system to develop a defense to the disease without introducing the disease itself to the body. Vaccines take advantage of the body's ability, via the immune system, to repel any micro or germ attacking it. When the body is attacked, the immune system will take some time to develop a defense to combat the disease germs, and if or when it shows up again, it will be ready to eliminate the threat. Vaccines give the immune system time to develop immunity to that particular germ. If the germ comes to the body again, it will be ready to instantly defend against the germ or disease.

Core Vaccines

Core vaccines are the vaccines that are recommended for all dogs and should be given starting as a puppy. These viral diseases are:

- **Rabies -** A disease that is always fatal in dogs. Vaccination is required by law in the United States. Not having this vaccination will not only cause your dog to die, but if the dog bites a human while diseased with rabies, the human will be quarantined and there is a possibility of death.
- **Distemper -** A highly contagious and fatal disease, especially for puppies. The most common affliction associated with this disease is seizures.
- **Parvovirus -** The most common viral disease for dogs. It is more common in puppies than in adult dogs. It is highly contagious and is spread by an infected dog's feces. The virus can live for months on shoes, clothes, carpets, and floors.
- **Adenovirus (canine hepatitis) -** Is a disease that may cause respiratory infection and kennel cough. It is spread through saliva, feces, urine, blood, or nasal discharge from an infected dog. The disease affects the liver and can be fatal in 30 percent of dogs who contract the disease if not vaccinated.

Noncore Vaccines

These vaccines are recommended based on your geological location and your dog's exposure risk to the disease in the environment. This category of vaccines is where some people prefer not to have their dog inoculated because the risk of over vaccination is dangerous to the dog's health. Some of the noncore vaccinations are.

- **Bordetella -** A bacteria that is the most common cause of tracheobronchitis or kennel cough. The disease is spread when your dog mixes with other dogs in large numbers,

in shows, parks, or kennel. If your dog is exposed to large number of dogs, you need to vaccinate every six months.
- **Lyme disease -** Caused by a bacteria carried by a black-legged tick found in every state in the US. This affects dogs that spend a lot of time outside.
- **Leptospirosis -** A bacterial infection when the bacteria penetrated the skin and spreads throughout the body by way of the bloodstream. It occurs in tropical and subtropical areas with wet environments such as swamps and marshes.
- **Canine influenza -** A respiratory virus discovered in 2004, highly contagious and rapidly spreads between dogs. Also known to cause kennel cough.

Vaccine Titers

A vaccine titer is a blood test that determines if there are any antibodies in the dog's blood for a specific disease. It's a tool for dog owners and vets to minimize the risk of unnecessary vaccination and to see if your dog is still protected from a previous vaccination. Some vaccinations given when the dog was a puppy can work for the rest of the dog's life. Cost of titer test run about the same as a vaccination.

Vaccine Toxic Ingredients

Most vaccine manufacturers do not list the ingredients and claim its proprietary information even if the dog has a reaction to the vaccine. There are many manufacturers of the same vaccine but different ingredients, and knowing what is in the vaccine would help avoid a reaction in your pet. Most rabies vaccines contain mercury. These additives with mercury are named thimerosal or thiomersal and merthiolate, to name a few. Mercury is a poison and is used as a preservative for the vaccine.

Vaccine Reaction

If your dog is a little lethargic or restless right after a vaccination, it is not something to worry about. The vaccine will stimulate the immune system and the dog will return to normal in a day or two. Reactions usually develop in small breeds and young dogs. Administering multiple vaccines at one time is also a trigger. Although uncommon, some dogs will react to a vaccination and medical attention is required immediately. The reaction to vaccines is one or more of the following symptoms:

- Swelling at the face and the injection point
- Difficulty breathing
- Hives
- Collapse
- Vomiting
- Loss of appetite
- Fever
- Diarrhea
- Seizures

Vaccine Dosage

Doses for dogs are all the same, 1ml. It's the same for a Chihuahua as it is for a Great Dane. Vaccines are used to stimulate the immune system and its inoculation is not based on weight.

Vaccine Recommendation

In 2011, the American Animal Hospital Association introduced a Canine Vaccination Guidelines, which updated recommendations for vaccination. A task force of veterinarians and professionals put together the guidelines and recommendations to establish a protocol, treatment, and procedure for vaccinations based on available scientific evidence, immunological principles, and expert consensus. The group contends that vaccination is the safest and most cost-effective means of infectious disease prevention available to date.

CHAPTER 18

Flea and Tick Prevention

Collars - Toxins in flea and tick collars are toxic to dogs and can bring on a seizure. The chemicals that are strong enough to annihilate pesky insects are strong enough to harm you and your dog. The Environmental Protection Agency (EPA) banned many of the pesticides used in flea and tick treatments from other household uses fifteen years ago, but overlooked them in pet products. Exposure to these toxic ingredients can cause birth defects, disruption of hormones, and cancer. The most dangerous among them can have a long-term impact on young children, impairing their neurological development.

To combat it, the EPA is calling for new labeling requirements including warnings, a listing of possible symptoms, better labeling instructions, dosage guidelines for consumers, and even possible restrictions of certain ingredients. No products are being banned, but Owens says EPA is not ruling out such drastic measures in the future.

Flea-fighting collars for dogs and puppies often harbor toxic chemicals that can mess with your body's hormones and even your nervous system. The highest-risk ingredients have been linked to cancer.

Check the active ingredient on the label; that is the pesticide used. Avoid anything with **propoxur** or **tetrachlorvinphos**—both have been identified by the EPA as likely carcinogens (meaning, there's a strong possibility that they cause cancer). **Amitraz** is another chemical sometimes used in flea collars. It's a known "developmental toxicant" that can, when pregnant women are exposed to it, result in low birth weights, birth defects, and biological and psychological problems that show up as the child grows.

Types of Collars

1. **High-frequency collar** - These work by sending out an ultrasonic sound wave that "scares" fleas away. Despite a number of positive reports, I remain slightly doubtful and haven't had much success with these electronic collars myself. However, I must admit that I haven't used them for very long, so if you have had any good (or bad) experience with them, please let me know so I can share it with others.
2. **Gas-based collar** - These create a gas-based toxin that repels fleas from your dog or cat. It kills fleas on contact, provided they actually come near the collar. In other words, it's not going to affect any fleas if they are not exposed to the limited area around your pet's neck. However, the good news is that fleas are not that intelligent and won't know about the gas (they cannot smell it or anything), so they may be exposed to it and "expire" on the spot!
3. **Absorption-based collar** - These also contain insecticide but instead of "floating around" your pet's fur to keep the fleas away, it actually gets absorbed into their skin. When its fleas' dinner time and they start nibbling on your pet, they are killed by the poison. However, exposure to this poison has left many wondering about their pets' safety. Is it really something to be concerned about?

Flea Powder - Used for parasite control and has a toxic chemical known as organochlorines. Check your flea collar brand for this chemical ingredients. Another chemical toxin called pyrethrin used to control skin parasites is also deadly and causes seizures. Powder on flea and tick collars gets everywhere. When tests were done on flea and tick collars, they looked at how much of the pesticides were leaching out of the flea collars and how much remain on a pet's coat after three days. One of the problems with powder is it spreads to furniture, bedding, toys, and your hands. Remember, this is a pesticide.

Flea and Tick Shampoos - It is recommended to avoid certain brands of flea and tick shampoo altogether because of their "high risk" ingredients. Chemicals in these shampoos are highly toxic.

Sprays - One of the active ingredients often found in these pest control sprays is **tetrachlorvinphos**, a suspected carcinogen that is toxic to the nervous system. Overexposure to this pesticide can cause nausea and vomiting and, in severe cases, seizures and respiratory paralysis. It can even be fatal. The NRDC warns that young children are particularly susceptible to it because of their relative inability to metabolize chemicals and their still-developing nervous systems.

The EPA underestimated the amount of exposure kids can have to household pets and allowed older pesticides with "bad track records" into the market.

Active ingredients **permethrin** and **piperonyl butoxide (PBO)** are "possible carcinogens," meaning researchers say there's a strong likelihood that they cause cancer. One study also linked prenatal exposure to PBO to delays in neurodevelopment.

Oral Medications (Pills) - An oral flea control medication can cause upset stomach and vomiting in some dogs. Remember that these are all insecticides made to kill insects. As with any oral medication, the dog bedding and carpeting need to be cleaned to remove any flea or flea eggs.

Over-the-counter oral medications for flea control include:

- Advantage
- Capstar
- Capguard
- Fastcaps
- Program Oral Suspension

Advantage

Advantage II is regarded as one of the better over-the-counter oral medications for fleas since it is highly effective and has very few side effects. It kills fleas, flea eggs, and larvae. As with most oral medications, it does not kill ticks.

Capstar

Capstar is an oral medication that usually takes within thirty minutes to kill fleas after ingestion. It works well with fleas, but does not affect ticks. One pill is effective for twenty-four hours, then another dose is required. Capstar comes in two strengths: one for small dogs and one for larger dogs.

Capguard

Capguard begins to kill fleas within thirty minutes. Side effects can be lethargy. vomiting trembling, and even seizures. This oral medication should not be used on dogs under twenty-five pounds or eight weeks old.

Fastcaps

Fastcaps has the same active ingredient as Capstar, and is effective thirty minutes after ingestion. Dosage is every twenty-four hours.

Program

Program is an oral medication that renders flea eggs unhatchable but does not kill the adult flea. It is given once a month to dogs older than six weeks.

Prescription oral medications for flea control include:

- Bravecto
- Comfortis
- Sentinel
- NexGard

Bravecto

Bravecto is an oral medication that works within hours and is good for twelve weeks of protection with a single dose. It also protects against ticks.

Comfortis

Comfortis is a beef-flavored chewable tablet, which makes it palatable to dogs. It takes effect within a half hour and has to be taken once a month. It kills adult fleas and destroys flea eggs and larvae. As with Capstar, it does not destroy active tick infections.

Sentinel

Sentinel is a combination flea and heartworm pill that does not kill fleas but stops their development. Sentinel contains milbemycin oxime, a medication that protects your pet from flea infections and prevents your dog from suffering from worm infections like heartworms, roundworms, hookworms, and whipworms. It is administered once a month.

NexGard

NexGard protects your dog against fleas and ticks with a beef-flavored chewy for up to one month. This is for dogs and puppies eight weeks of age and older.

Alternatives to Flea and Tick Products

If it's prevention you're looking for here (and not treatment for an existing flea or tick problem), chemicals are not necessarily needed. Use a fine-tooth flea comb on your pet daily and wash their bedding in hot, soapy water every week.

The risk associated with spot-on treatments is there is simply no chemical-based pest control pill, dip, solution, shampoo, or collar that has no potential side effects.

Just because a compound is applied to or worn on your pet's fur does not mean it's safe. Remember: what goes **on** your pet goes **in** your pet, by absorption through the skin or ingestion during grooming.

Fleas, ticks, mosquitoes, and other parasites feed first on unhealthy animals. So the goal of preventive pest control is to bring your dog or cat to optimal health, which will make them naturally more resilient and less attractive to parasites.

- Essential oil sprays containing lavender, peppermint, geranium, lemongrass, or citronella can be very effective as parasite deterrents. You need to purchase a preblended product or work with an animal aroma therapist to make sure you're using safe oils at the correct concentration as dog and cat doses are different.

- Cedar oil is a long-recognized flea eradicator, and products exist that are specially formulated for cats and dogs.
- Natural, food-grade diatomaceous earth helps to remove fleas and ticks from your pet's body.
- Fresh garlic can be given to dogs and cats to prevent internal as well as external parasites. Work with your vet to determine a safe amount for your pet's body weight.
- Herbal flea powder can be made from eucalyptus, rosemary, lemon, clary sage, peppermint, palmarosa, lavender, and fennel. This concoction will repel fleas but not kill them. Another is an essential oil flea powder using cedar, pine, niaouli, and baking soda.

Cleanliness and the Living Environment

The place where your dog lives, their environment is the place where the flea makes its home. So it is extremely important to constantly clean the living area. Even though flea eggs can remain dormant for months if they have to, they normally hatch every three days. Vacuuming the area around the dog's bedding and washing the bedding twice a week can eliminate the flea eggs, larvae, and pupae. Although a flea is on a dog, they live mainly on your pet's bedding. Once you have sanitized the dog's bedding, apply a small amount of diatomaceous earth (DE) around the area. It may feel like talcum powder, but to a flea its razor-sharp glass and easily cuts the flea's shell. It's harmless to pets and humans. Placing the DE dust in cracks and crevices where a flea may hide is a natural and not at all toxic. Note that the DE used for pest control is not the same as the DE used in pool filters. Salt is another natural ingredient that kills flea eggs by dehydrating them.

CHAPTER 19

Medications and Drugs

Although some veterinarians do use human drugs for dogs with certain ailments, most medications are not safe for canines. Please consult your veterinarian before giving any over-the-counter medications for pain.

NSAIDs

Nonsteroidal anti-inflammatory drugs are a common household drug. This class of drug is found over-the-counter, like ibuprofen, naproxen, and others. Some of the brands include Motrin, Advil, and Aleve. Ingestion of even small amounts of ibuprofen can lead to vomiting and diarrhea as well as gastric ulceration, bleeding, and perforation. At high-enough concentrations, it can cause permanent kidney damage and affect the central nervous system leading to seizures, inability to walk, coma, and death. Treatment of the dog includes decontamination through emesis, prevention and treatment of gastric ulceration, renal failure, and CNS effects. Common therapies will include inducing vomiting, giving activated charcoal, GI protectants such as omeprazole, carafate, misoprostol, and IV fluid therapy. Blood will also be monitored to check kidney function. The prognosis is good if the patient is treated immediately after ingestion. Just one or two pills (depending on the dog's weight) of these medications can cause kidney failure and seizures.

Acetaminophen

Tylenol, Percoset, aspirin-free Excedrin are common and popular over-the-counter pain, cold and flu medication. Dog owners too often medicate their dogs with a toxic dose of these medicines without consulting a veterinarian first, or the dog finds a pill accidently dropped on the floor. Once ingested, it takes thirty minutes to get into the bloodstream and damage the liver. A dog taking a pill can have severe liver failure and damage to the red blood cells. The symptoms of acetaminophen toxicity in dogs include lethargy, decreased appetite, swollen face, difficulty breathing, vomiting, hypothermia (lower body temperature), gray gums, jaundice, coma, and death.

Since acetaminophen can be absorbed so quickly, the first thing is prompt medical attention from an emergency animal hospital or veterinarian since this can be fatal. The first treatment is to induce vomiting to remove as much of the drug from the stomach before it is absorbed. A veterinarian will use liquid-activated charcoal to absorb the toxin from the stomach and intestines. The vet may also use a specific antidotal medication, like N-acetylcysteine or NAC (Mucomyst), that will metabolize the toxic drug in the liver and eliminate it from the body. The dog may need a blood transfusion.

The main toxicity to a dog is the damage to the liver and the inability of blood to carry oxygen. Survival is based on how quickly the dog gets to a hospital or vet for treatment following ingestion of a toxic amount of acetaminophen. If the liver is damaged beyond repair, the result may be death despite treatment. If your dog has acetaminophen toxicity, the only thing you can do is get to a hospital or vet as soon as possible. If your dog manages to survive acetaminophen toxicity, permanent liver damage may occur and the dog may need special diets and lifetime medications to counteract the liver damage.

The bottom line is, do not give any medications to a dog without the approval of your veterinarian.

Pseudoephedrine (and Other Nasal Decongestants)

Depending on the circumstances of exposure, pseudoephedrine can be very harmful or even deadly to pets, and therefore we would not advise giving it to your dog. Decongestants are frequently found in products that contain antihistamines. If your veterinarian has prescribed an antihistamine, please read the label carefully to be sure that the only active ingredient is the one your veterinarian recommends.

Benzodiazepine

A sleep aid, commonly sold as Lunesta, Xanax, Ambien, and Klonopin, that is toxic and causes slowed breathing and listlessness. Cholesterol-lowering drugs known as statins can cause serious problems in dogs if there is a large quantity or taken over a period of time.

Diphenhydramine Hydrochloride

Also known as Benadryl, it is an antihistamine that is commonly used to treat canine allergies. Although not licensed for veterinary use, it is commonly used in that field. Some dogs may be allergic to this drug and react with a seizure.

Tramadol

With the brand name known as Ultram, it is a pain reliever and is sometimes prescribed by vets. If the dose is too high, the dog will have a seizure.

Adderall

It is an attention deficit hyperactivity disorder (ADHD) drug used in children as a sedative. It has the opposite effect in dogs, wherein it stimulates them, causing high heart rates, high body temperature, and seizures.

Amphetamine

Desoxyn and Dexedrine are also ADHD drugs. Although not approved for dogs, some vets use this drug. A pill for human use can cause overstimulation of the dog's nervous system, causing heavy panting, shaking aggression, and seizure.

Antidepressants

Known as duloxetine or venlafaxine, they are sold as Cymbalta or Effexor. When ingested by dogs, they can cause tremors and seizures.

Medications that may be safe for people can be fatal to dogs. Also, make sure that all medications are kept out of the reach of inquisitive dogs. Keeping medicine safely stored away can prevent many tragedies. The most common symptoms that you may notice in pets suffering from acetaminophen toxicity include: brownish gray-colored gums, labored breathing, swollen face, neck, or limbs, hypothermia (reduced body temperature), vomiting, jaundice (yellowish color to skin, whites of eyes) due to liver damage, and coma.

Canine Medications

Some medications are designed for dogs, but can be toxic and can cause seizures.

Ivermectin is a parasiticide medicine given to dogs for the prevention of heartworm and other internal parasites. Some dogs are inherently sensitive to the drug. Also, the dosage is very important to keep it below the toxic level.

Fluoroquinolone is a common antibiotic known as Baytril, Orbax, Cipro, and Zeniquin. These are prescribed for dogs in the treatment of skin, bladder, ear, kidneys, and other ailments. There is a risk of joint damage causing the dog to become lame and worse a deadly condition known as aortic aneurysm.

Isoniazid is a human antituberculosis drug that is also used by veterinarians to treat canine infections with certain strains of bacteria. Even in low dosage, the drug can be toxic and can cause coma, seizures, and death.

Lamotrigine (Lamictal) is another drug used to treat bipolar disorder in humans. As with other human drugs, even at low dosage the drug can be toxic to certain dog breeds.

Phenylbutazone is an anti-inflammatory medication for dogs to alleviate pain and inflammation in limbs due to fractures or arthritis. This drug requires close monitoring due to the adverse side effects to the kidneys and liver from the suppression of white blood cells and anemia.

Corticosteroid is a type of steroid that is used for canine allergies or joint pain. There are many serious side effects and should be used as a last resort.

Phenylpropanolamine (Proin) is a drug prescribed for urinary incontinence in older dogs, usually females. The most common side effect is elevated heart rate, restlessness, and high blood pressure. This drug can cause seizures in dogs as well as strokes.

Famotidine (Pepcid AC) is used to reduce the amount of stomach acid being produced. Used by most vets, some dogs develop serious side effects from it, including trouble breathing and swelling of the tongue, lips, or face.

Any medications with the potential to cause hypoglycemia such as sulfonylureas and diabetic medications can all cause seizures in dogs.

Most dogs are curious over every little thing they find. They smell it and it goes into their mouth. If you have any prescription medication or drug, be sure that they are out of reach of your pet. Never leave pills on the counter or pill bottles open where your dog can reach them. If you drop a pill, pick it up immediately. Never give a pill to your dog unless prescribed by your veterinarian. If your dog has ingested a pill not prescribed to them, call your vet immediately.

Illicit Drugs

The Illicit drugs listed here are all toxic and poisonous to dogs and will cause seizures:
Cocaine
Amphetamines
Cannabis
Synthetic cannabinoids

CHAPTER 20

What Foods Are Toxic to Dogs

There are foods that are edible for humans, but are toxic and pose a hazard to dogs. A dog's metabolism, the breakdown of foods, is different than humans' and may cause upset stomachs and in other cases cause seizures and death. Listed here are foods that are toxic and dangerous to dogs.

Alcohol, which contains ethanol, is toxic and even fatal for dogs. Over time, excessive alcohol can cause liver, kidney, and nervous system damage. Dogs can also get alcohol by infesting fermented food. Symptoms (like humans) are drowsiness, loss of coordination, and slow movements. Enough alcohol and the dog will drop their blood sugar levels and have a seizure.

Apple seeds – Although apples are a good source of fiber and vitamins, the apple seeds contain a form of cyanide, which is a poison that prevents the blood from carrying oxygen throughout the body. Core the apple before giving them to your dog.

Avocado – Avocados contain a toxin called persin, which can cause an upset stomach in a dog, but contrary to some it is not toxic to dogs.

Baby food – Some baby food have onion powder in them, which can be toxic, but baby food is low in nutrients for a dog's diet.

Cooked bones – Cooked chicken bones become brittle and will splinter when chewed by a dog. When swallowed, they can puncture the throat or stomach. Raw bones are safe, nutritional, and clean the dog's teeth.

Candy and chewing gum – Many gum and candies use xylitol, an artificial sweetener. When ingested, it causes a surge in insulin in the body, resulting in a drop in blood sugar that can damage the liver and can cause kidney failure and/or a seizure.

Cat food – Cat food is higher in fat with extra protein for a cat's dietary needs. It also affects the gastrointestinal tract of a dog, causing diarrhea, vomiting, and pancreatitis.

Chocolate, coffee, and caffeine – There are many sources of caffeine in your home: tea, coffee, soda, energy drinks, diet pills, and more. When a pet ingests caffeine, it can result in an upset stomach to seizures, depending on the intake and weight of the dog. Chocolate contains a dangerous toxin called theobromine. Similar to caffeine, dogs are very sensitive to it, but the fat and sugar involved is detrimental to a dog's pancreas.

Citrus – The ASPCA considers oranges, lemons, limes, and grapefruit to be toxic to dogs, with the seeds, leaves, and skin of the citrus the most dangerous parts. Ingestion of a small amount will cause an upset stomach, and larger amounts will cause vomiting, depression, diarrhea, and photosensitivity.

Citrus oil extracts – Used in many household products, including shampoos, insecticides, cleaners, and perfumes. Usually ingested by a young puppy, citrus oil can cause drooling, weakness, hypothermia, low blood pressure, and depression. A vet may flush the stomach or use activated charcoal to treat it.

Coconut and coconut oil – Coconut pulp and coconut milk can be ingested by a dog but contain oils that could upset the stomach and cause diarrhea.

Corn on the cob – The corn itself is not dangerous to a dog. In fact, it contains essential fatty acids, protein, and antioxidants. The real problem is if a part of a cob gets stuck in the intestines and causes an obstruction. This means a trip to the vet and surgery.

Fat trimmings – A small amount of steak fat trimmed from meat, both cooked and uncooked, given occasionally will not hurt your dog, but it is better to give your dog lean meat. Too much fat and your dog can develop pancreatitis.

Fish – Fish is a great source of omega-3 fatty acids, which dogs need for a healthy body. Salmon fish that are infected with a parasite can be extremely dangerous and fatal to a dog if it is eaten raw. Cooking the salmon thoroughly will kill the parasite and make it safe for your dog.

Garlic – There is a controversy surrounding garlic as to if it's beneficial to dogs or if it's toxic to dogs. The fact is, it is good for your dog *in small amounts*. In large amounts, garlic is toxic. Garlic has a compound called thiosulfate, which causes damage to the red blood cells in the body. The average clove of garlic in the grocery store is 3 to 7 grams. The amount to be toxic in a dog is 15 to 30 grams. But there are some dogs that are sensitive to garlic and that would cause problems. Symptoms include diarrhea, vomiting, loss of appetite, and abdominal pain.

Grapes and raisins – No one knows what the toxic substance is in grapes and raisins, but consuming them can cause lethargy, diarrhea, vomiting, and then kidney failure. Do not feed grapes and raisins to dogs.

Hops are used in brewing beer and also used as cattle food. Hops are very toxic to dogs and cause hyperthermia. Small amounts can cause fever, severe panting, and rapid heartbeat. The dog will need a veterinarian to be treated for hop toxicity. Very few dogs survive this poison.

Human vitamins – Most human vitamins are safe to give dogs as long as the weight ratio between dogs and humans is understood and they are free of iron and zinc, both of which are toxic to dogs. Also, vitamin A and D are toxic if given too much of a dose. It is best to stick with canine vitamins.

Liver is a very high nutritional meat to give to your dog. It has a good source of protein, vitamin A, good fatty acids, and other nutrients. The problem is the liver is so high in vitamin A that your dog can overdose. An overdose can lead to digestive problems, weakness, and bone spurs. Only small portions twice a week.

Macadamia nuts – Although the macadamia nut is very toxic to a dog, the exact cause of the poison is not known. The sensitivity is different in each dog, and signs show up after twelve hours. The most common is the inability to walk with the hind legs, vomiting, tremors, and high temperature. Your vet may administer charcoal to absorb any nuts in the digestive tract, with the dog returning to normal after twenty-four hours.

Marijuana – Dogs that usually ingest marijuana usually get ahold of a cookie laced with it since it's legal in many states. A small amount won't hurt your dog, but a large amount can cause lethargy, low heart rate, low blood pressure, and seizures.

Milk and dairy products – Most dogs are lactose intolerant, and this can cause diarrhea, gas, or vomiting. But dairy items low in lactose, like cheese and cottage cheese, served in small amounts are tolerable.

Mushrooms - There is some benefits to edible mushrooms that you get at the market or even mushroom extracts, but in some dogs, the result is diarrhea and vomiting. Never let a pet eat wild mushrooms, unless you're an expert on mushrooms.

Nuts – Many commonly eaten nuts are toxic to dogs. These include almonds, walnuts, pistachios, macadamia, and pecans. All nuts are high in fat, and if dogs ingest enough, they can develop pancreatitis. Also, dogs cannot digest fats well, so they develop digestive blockages, which can be painful and require surgery.

Onions and chives – Like garlic, onion contains thiosulpate, a toxin that causes anemia in dogs, damages the red blood cells, and can be fatal. Symptoms are loss of appetite and lethargy. In higher amounts consumed, the symptoms are heavy panting, abdominal pain, vomiting, diarrhea, increased heart rate, and seizure.

Persimmons are a good source of iron and potassium and are not toxic to dogs. However, if your dog consumes a couple of fruits, it will be like a laxative. The seeds are large and could be lodged in the intestine, causing serious problems.

Peaches are not toxic and are good for your dog. The main problem is the pit. If chewed and swallowed by a dog, its sharp edges can cut the lining of the intestines, and if the stone was chewed and broken up, it contains cyanide. Cyanide is also in the tree leaves and stems.

Plums – Like peaches, plums are not toxic to dogs, but the pit contains cyanide and is poisonous, plus the pit could get stuck in the intestines and cause a blockage.

Rhubarb – The stalk of the rhubarb is not toxic to dogs and even has a laxative effect on dogs. The problem is the rhubarb leaves, which can be harmful if ingested. The leaves are very bitter, so dogs seldom eat them.

Raw eggs – The problem with raw eggs are that the enzymes in the raw eggs interfere with the absorption of biotin, a vitamin B complex. Also, raw eggs can have salmonella bacteria that can cause fever, diarrhea, and vomiting, and can be fatal. Cooking eggs are a better alternative.

Raw fish is good for a dog because of the omega-3 benefits that a dog can get from fish. The big three problems are tapeworms, roundworms, and fluke found in raw fish.

Raw/undercooked meat and bones – With raw meat and bones, you are accepting the risk that the meat or bones are not contaminated with roundworm, salmonella, E. coli, and other diseases. If you insist on a raw-meat diet, get your meat from a local butcher, with all the regulations and sanitation in place, and make sure it's balanced with vegetables.

Raw hide treats – Dogs love to chew and one of the things we give them to satisfy this craving is raw hide treats. Made from a cow or pig, these raw hides are cleaned and flavored but are not cooked. Although they are great for cleaning the teeth of a dog, there are concerns that some large piece can break off, lodge in the digestive tract, and choke your dog, or the raw hide that comes from outside the United States, particularly China, could be contaminated with salmonella or E. coli.

Salt – Salt should not be given to dogs because all their sodium (salt) requirements are taken care of from the food they eat. Too much salt can cause vomiting, diarrhea, lethargy, excessive thirst, muscle spasms, damage to the kidneys, brain swelling, seizures, and death. Treatments include IV fluids for dehydration.

Spices – The spices to avoid, other than the one previously addressed, are:

- **nutmeg**
- **cocoa powder**

Nutmeg contains a toxin called myristicin, and even a small amount is a serious toxin enough to cause hallucinations, disorientation, high blood pressure, abdominal pain, and seizures.

Cocoa powder – Since cocoa powder is a chocolate, it contains theobromine, a caffeine-related toxin to dogs. Symptoms are abdominal pain, fever, increased heart rate, and possibly a seizure.

Sugar – Dogs can be affected just like humans with sugar intake. Diabetes, obesity, and dental problems are the problems with extra sugar intake. Dogs get plenty of sugar from regular dog food and occasional fruit in its diet.

Tobacco – Along with tobacco are a number of items with nicotine in them that do the same thing. Besides cigarettes, there are cigar butts, nicotine patch, nicotine gum, e-cigarette fluid, and chewing tobacco. Dogs will show signs of poisoning within an hour of ingestion. Symptoms are fast heart rate, high blood pressure, vomiting, diarrhea, drooling, trembling, constricted pupils, seizures, and death.

Xylitol is a sugar substitute found in gum, candy, toothpaste, and baked goods that is safe for people but highly toxic to dogs. Within fifteen minutes of ingestion, the dog's symptoms are a drop in blood pressure, vomiting, seizures, and liver damage.

Yeast dough – Yeast dough can rise and cause gas to accumulate in your pet's digestive system. This can be painful and can cause the stomach to bloat and potentially twist it, becoming a life-threatening emergency. The yeast produces ethanol as a by-product, and a dog ingesting raw bread dough can cause drunkenness.

Food Additives

Listed below are some of the food additives that are harmful to dogs:

Foods with ethoxyquin, BHA, or BHT Treats with ethoxyquin, BHA, or BHT

MSG (sometimes called natural flavoring, smoke flavoring, etc.)

Forgo salty treats. Foods and treats with a lot of salt can actually cause your dog to have a seizure if they are on potassium bromide, so cut them out of the diet.

While these don't fall in a particular category above, you will want to avoid them as well:

Old food – You don't like old and moldy food, so what makes you think your dog will? The bacteria in spoiled food contain all sorts of toxins that can be damaging to your dog's health. Feed them the freshest and best dog-approved food only!

Leftovers – I know it's difficult to keep your dog from feasting on your dinner leftovers after they have had to sit there and watch you eat it all in front of them. But the fact is that if you feed them leftovers regularly, they won't be getting a proper diet. If you do give them table scraps, make sure to take out any bones and trim down the fat.

Check the ingredients – Bottom line is, be sure to know what is in the food you're giving your dog. The items from the list above should definitely not be in there. You would be surprised at how many foods contain sugar and caffeine that you would not expect to without first checking the ingredient list.

Human snacks – Chips, pretzels, and popcorn can contain garlic and onion powder, and cookies may contain raisins, chocolate, or macadamia nuts, etc. Bottom line: there's a reason why there are food and treats made especially for dogs.

Chapter 21

Plants

It is impossible to capture the thousands of plant varieties, and this list does not represent all toxic plants that may cause seizures. Your dog may also have an allergy or sensitivity to some of these plants. Note that some of these plants do not cause seizures, but the poisons have an effect on the dogs' immune system and neurological system, and prolonged exposure to poisonous plants will cause seizures if not corrected.

If you suspect your dog is poisoned, call a veterinarian or a dog poison hotline immediately. If the poison just occured, vomiting is the best method to get rid as much toxic from the poison as possible. To induce vomiting, give your dog 3 percent solution of hydrogen peroxide (1 teaspoon per 10 pounds of body weight). Repeat every fifteen minutes for a maximum of three times. In any case, if you experience any of these plant poisonings, see a veterinarian immediately.

A

Aconite – is toxic if eaten, and can cause nausea and vomiting. It may also affect cardiac function—increased heart rate.

African Wonder Tree – Leaves may contain ricin—a toxic to dogs; it can also cause loss of appetite, excessive thirst, weakness, colic, trembling, sweating, loss of coordination, difficulty in breathing, depression, bloody diarrhea, seizures, and death.

Aloe Vera – **(May cause)** vomiting, lethargy, and diarrhea. The gel is considered edible to humans.

Amaryllis – Especially popular around Easter, the lovely amaryllis is also poisonous to dogs. Its toxins can cause vomiting, depression, diarrhea, abdominal pain, hypersalivation, anorexia, and tremors to dogs.

American Holly – is toxic if eaten, and may cause nausea and vomiting.

Toxin contains saponins.

American Mandrake – **can cause** vomiting, diarrhea, lethargy, panting, coma (rare), dermal – redness, and skin ulcers.

American Yew – **Signs of poisoning are** tremors, difficulty breathing, vomiting, seizures, and sudden death from acute heart failure.

Andromeda Japonica – Signs **of poisoning** are vomiting, diarrhea, weakness, and cardiac failure.

Angels Trumpets – is toxic if eaten, and can cause nausea and vomiting.

Angels Wings – can result in upset stomach, oral irritation, asphyxiation, tremors, seizures, loss of balance, and can be fatal.

Anemone – Signs of poisoning are vomiting, diarrhea, weakness, and cardiac failure.

Apple – **its** seeds contain cyanide, and has varied toxic effects.

Apple Leaf Croton – its bark, root, and sap are toxic to dogs. If chewed or swallowed, these chemicals can cause swelling and blistering in the mouth; if enough is ingested, it can also cause vomiting and diarrhea. The sap can also cause an eczema–like reaction when it comes in contact with the skin. The symptoms are abdominal pain, mouth blisters, diarrhea, eczema, eye irritation, nausea, skin irritation, and vomiting.

Apricot – **the** kernels contain cyanide, and can be fatal.

Arbovitae – is harmful if eaten in quantity, and may cause skin allergy

Arrowhead vine –Signs of poisoning **are o**ral irritation, pain, swelling of mouth, tongue, and lips, excessive drooling, vomiting, and difficulty in swallowing.

Arrow grasses – (leaves)

Asian Lily – **can cause** excessive drooling, nausea, diarrhea, decreased heart rate, cardiac arrhythmia, and seizure.

Asparagus Fern – contains a wide variety of poisons resulting to a large range of symptoms.

Atropa belladonna – is one of the most toxic plants; the roots are the most deadly, but any part of it is deadly including the sweet purple–black berries. Symptoms of poisoning are excessive salivation, lack of appetite, vomiting, diarrhea, drowsiness, dilated pupils, confusion, convulsions, weakness, slow breathing, slow heart rate and respiratory failure.

Australian Nut (Macadamia nut) – may cause depression, hyperthermia, weakness, muscular stiffness, vomiting, tremors, and increased heart rate.

Autumn Crocus – can cause an intense burning sensation in the mouth, vomiting, diarrhea, seizures, liver and kidney damage, and even heart arrhythmias. Although the entire plant is considered toxic to dogs, the toxicity is highest in the bulbs of the plant, and can be fatal.

Avocado – **may cause** diarrhea, vomiting, labored breathing, and can be fatal.

Azalea – A member of the widely toxic genus rhododendron, the azalea is found in many varieties all over the United States, and is commonly used as an ornamental flowering shrub in landscaping. It may cause nausea, vomiting, depression, difficulty in breathing, and coma.

B

Baby's Breath – causes a mild toxic reaction paired with vomiting, diarrhea, anorexia, lethargy, and depression.

Bay Laural – Signs of poisoning are vomiting and diarrhea. Large ingestion of whole leaves can cause obstruction; the principal toxin is eugenol.

Balsem Pair – ingestion may result to vomiting, diarrhea, and pain in the stomach.

Baneberry – Baneberry is a wildflower found in North America. It is known for its toxic berries which can be in glossy red or white. Ingestion of only a few berries can be fatal. Symptoms of poisoning are irritation around the mouth and throat, vomiting, diarrhea, and abdominal pain.

Barilla – Leaves and stems are toxic. Signs of poisoning are vomiting and diarrhea.

Bead Tree – Signs of poisoning are diarrhea, vomiting, salivation, depression, weakness, and seizures. Ripe fruit or berries are most toxic but the bark, leaves, and flowers are toxic too.

Bergamot Orange – **Signs** of poisoning **are** vomiting, diarrhea, depression, and potential photosensitivity or dermatitis.

Begonia – may result in kidney failure, vomiting, and salivation in dogs/cats. The most toxic part is underground.

Bird of Paradise – can cause oral irritation, intense burning, irritation of mouth, tongue, and lips, excessive drooling, vomiting, diarrhea, difficulty swallowing, and loss of coordination is possible. Gastrointestinal tract may be affected by the plant toxins.

Bittersweet, American/Waxwork – is toxic if eaten, and can cause nausea, vomitin, and seizures.

Bittersweet European – is toxic if eaten, and can cause nausea and vomiting.

Black Cherry – the stems, leaves, and seeds contain cyanide; it is particularly toxic in the process of wilting. It can cause brick red mucous membranes, dilated pupils, difficulty in breathing, panting, and shock.

Black Locust – All parts of the plant is toxic with the seeds containing the highest concentration of toxins. Symptoms of poisoning include depression, weakness, diarrhea, vomiting, convulsions, and respiratory distress.

Black Walnuts – Dropping from black walnut trees by the thousands, the nuts themselves don't contain anything that can harm your dog. But once they start to decompose, they grow molds that <u>can cause tremors and seizures</u>. If you have one of these trees in your yard, and your dog seems to be attracted to the nuts, it might be a good idea to rake them up on a regular basis.

Bleeding Heart – is poisonous in large amounts, contains convulsants, and may also cause dermatitis.

Bloodroot – can cause nausea, vomiting, tiredness, vertigo, and dizziness—eventually, organ failure.

Bluebell – can be harmful if eaten in quantity.

Bobbins – Signs of poisoning are oral irritation, intense burning and irritation of mouth, tongue, and lips, excessive drooling, vomiting, and difficulty in swallowing.

Bog Laurel – Signs of poisoning are vomiting, diarrhea, weakness, and cardiac failure.

Borage – Signs of poisoning are vomiting, diarrhea, dermatitis.

Boston ivy – can result in mouth swelling, respiratory issues, gastrointestinal/stomach upset, and you can have difficulty in swallowing.

Boxwood – can cause upset stomach, heart failure, excitability or lethargy, and may also cause dermatitis.

Bracken – may cause thiamine deficiency, acute hemorrhagic syndrome, blindness, and tumors.

Bread and Butter Plant – Signs of poisoning are vomiting, diarrhea, depression, anorexia, occasionally bloody diarrhea, or vomiting.

Broom – Ingestion results in vomiting, abdominal discomfort, weakness, loss of coordination, and possible increased heart rate.

Buckeye (including nuts) – can be harmful if eaten in quantity.

Buckwheat – Sign of poisoning is photosensitization which may result in sunburn or dermatitis

Buddist Pine – Signs of poisoning are vomiting and diarrhea.

Burning Bush – can be toxic if eaten, and may cause nausea, vomiting, and skin allergy.

Buttercup – its juice may severely injure digestive system, and may also cause dermatitis.

Butterfly Iris – can result in salivation, vomiting, drooling, lethargy, and diarrhea. The highest concentration is in rhizomes.

C

Caladium – can result in oral irritation, pain and swelling of mouth, tongue, and lips, excessive drooling, vomiting, and difficulty in swallowing.

Calico Bush – is harmful if eaten in quantity.

Calla Lily – can result in oral irritation, intense burning and irritation of mouth, tongue and lips, excessive drooling, vomiting, and difficulty in swallowing

Cape Jasmine – can result in mild vomiting and/or diarrhea and hives.

Caraway – can result in mild vomiting and diarrhea.

Cardinal Flower – can result in depression, diarrhea, vomiting, excessive salivation, abdominal pain, and heart rhythm disturbances.

Castor Bean – This ornamental tropical plant, also used as a crop for castor oil, contains the toxic protein ricin. At the least, eating this plant can burn a dog's mouth and throat; it can lead to excessive thirst, vomiting and diarrhea, but ingestion of even an ounce of seeds can be lethal.

Ceriman – causes oral irritation, pain and swelling of mouth, tongue, and lips, excessive drooling, vomiting (not horses), difficulty in swallowing, and diarrhea if eaten. It may also cause dermatitis.

Chamomile – causes contact dermatitis, vomiting, diarrhea, anorexia, allergic reactions. Its long-term use can lead to bleeding tendencies.

Chandelier Plant – can result in vomiting, diarrhea, and abnormal heart rhythm.

Cherry – its kernels contain cyanide.

Cherry Laurel – is harmful if eaten in quantity.

Chinaberry Tree – may result in diarrhea, vomiting, salivation, depression, weakness, and seizures. Ripe fruit/berries are most toxic but bark, leaves, and flowers are toxic too.

Chinese Evergreen – may result in oral irritation, pain and swelling of mouth, tongue, and lips, excessive drooling, vomiting, and difficulty in swallowing.

Chinese Jade – can cause vomiting and tremors.

Chives – can cause vomiting, breakdown of red blood cells (hemolytic anemia and Heinz body anemia), blood in urine, weakness, high heart rate, and panting.

Choke Cherry – Stems, leaves, and seeds contain cyanide; it is particularly toxic in the process of wilting, and may result in brick red mucous membranes, dilated pupils, difficulty in breathing, panting, and shock.

Christmas Rose – is harmful if eaten in quantity.

Chrysanthemum – may cause dermatitis.

Cineraria – All the plant is toxic. Symptoms of poisoning are weakness, drowsiness, yawning, chewing, loss of coordination, diarrhea, and vomiting,

Clematis – Gastrointestinal tract and nervous system are affected by this plant's toxins, and may cause dermatitis.

Climbing Bittersweet – may cause weakness, convulsions, and gastroenteritis resulting to vomiting and diarrhea)

Climbing Lily – can cause bloody vomiting, diarrhea, shock, multi-organ damage, and bone marrow suppression.

Climbing Nightshade – commonly results in vomiting and diarrhea, and may sometimes cause drowsiness, low blood pressure, and low heart rate.

Cocoa husks or mulch – Similar toxic effects to that of chocolate –

hyperactivity, increased heart rate. Can kill if enough is eaten.

Coffee Tree – can cause contact dermatitis, vomiting, anorexia, and depression.

Corn Plant – can cause vomiting (with blood, occasionally), depression, anorexia, and hypersalivation.

Crocus – Symptoms of poisoning are drooling, vomiting, diarrhea, seizure, and may lead to death.

Croton – Symptoms of poisoning are vomiting, diarrhea, abdominal pain, blisters in mouth, eczema, eye irritation, and nausea.

Crown vetch – Symptoms of poisoning are vomiting, diarrhea, and abdominal pain.

Crowfoot – Symptoms of poisoning are vomiting, diarrhea, and abdominal pain.

Cycads – may result in vomiting (may be bloody), dark stools, jaundice, increased thirst, bloody diarrhea, bruising, liver failure, and death. One to two seeds can be fatal already.

Cyclamen – also known as Sowbread, the cyclamen is a common household flowering plant with poisonous properties (i.e., terpenoids) to dogs. It can cause oral irritation, vomiting, diarrhea, heart abnormalities, seizures, and death.

D

Daffodils – Among the first blooms to herald the arrival of spring, daffodils are a cheerful addition to the garden, but they contain poisonous alkaloids that can cause vomiting, excessive salivation, diarrhea, convulsions, tremors, and heart problems. The bulbs are the most dangerous part of the plant.

Daphne – Gastrointestinal tract and kidneys may be affected, and it may cause dermatitis.

Dahlia – may result in mild gastrointestinal signs and mild dermatitis.

Datura – is also called Jemsom weed and is very toxic. Symptoms of poisoning include vomiting, diarrhea, abdominal pain, asthenia, drowsiness, stupor, confusion, dilated pupils, and inability to eliminate.

Daisy – may cause vomiting, diarrhea, hypersalivation, in loss of coordination, and dermatitis.

Deadly Nightshade – is toxic if eaten, and may cause nausea and vomiting.

Delphinium – is also known as Larkspurs. Symptoms of poisoning include drooling, vomiting, constipation, abdominal pain, and slow heart rate.

Desert Azalea (Desert Rose) – can cause vomiting, diarrhea, anorexia, depression, irregular heartbeat, and death.

Devil's Backbone – may result in vomiting, diarrhea, and abnormal heart rhythm.

Devil's Fig – is harmful if eaten in quantity.

Devil's Ivy – may cause oral irritation, pain and swelling of mouth, tongue, and lips, excessive drooling, vomiting (not horses), and difficulty in swallowing.

Dieffenbachia – is also called Dumb Cane, and can cause diarrhea and oral irritation if eaten. It may also cause dermatitis, tremors, seizures, loss of balance, asphyxiation; it can be fatal. With its broad variegated leaves, the dieffenbachia is often recommended as an ideal houseplant for natural air purification.

Dock – may cause kidney failure, tremors, and salivation.

Dog Daisy – may result in increased urination, vomiting, diarrhea, and dermatitis.

Dog Hobble – can cause vomiting, diarrhea, depression, cardiovascular collapse, hypersalivation, weakness, coma, low blood pressure, and death. Ingestion of a few leaves can cause serious problems too.

Dogbane Hemp – may result in diarrhea (possibly with blood), slow heart rate, and weakness.

Dracaena – may cause vomiting (occasionally with blood), depression, anorexia, and hypersalivation.

Dragon tree – can cause diarrhea and vomiting.

Dumb Cane – *(See Dieffenbachia)*

Dwarf Moring Glory – is harmful if eaten in quantity.

Dwarf Poinciana – can cause vomiting and diarrhea.

E

Easter Lily – Especially poisonous to cats.

Easter Rose – can cause drooling, abdominal pain, diarrhea, colic, and depression.

Eastern Star – can cause vomiting and dermatitis.

Echium – is harmful if eaten in quantity, and may cause skin allergy.

Elder – Symptoms of poisoning are vomiting, diarrhea, and nausea— resulting in organ failure and death.

Elderberry – can cause nausea and vomiting.

Elephant Ears – can cause intense burning, irritation, and swelling of the mouth and throat. If tongue swells enough to block air passage, it can be fatal.

Emerald Feather – may cause allergic dermatitis with repeated dermal exposure. Berry ingestion could result in gastric upset including vomiting, abdominal pain, or diarrhea.

English Holly – can cause vomiting, diarrhea, and depression. Leaves and berries are low toxicity.

English Ivy – Gastrointestinal tract is affected. It may cause dermatitis.

English Yew – can cause tremors, difficulty in breathing, vomiting, seizures (in dogs), and sudden death from acute heart failure.

Epazote – is an essential oil, and can cause vomiting, and diarrhea (with ingestion of concentrated oils).

Eucalyptus – is an essential oil, and can cause salivation, vomiting, diarrhea, depression, and weakness.

European Bittersweet – can cause vomiting, diarrhea – common. Drowsiness, low blood pressure, low heart rate.

European Spindle – is harmful if eaten in quantity.

Everlasting Pea – Signs of poisoning are weakness, lethargy, pacing, head pressing, tremors, seizures, and can possibly lead to death.

Exotica – Signs of poisoning are oral irritation, intense burning and irritation of mouth, tongue, and lips, excessive drooling, vomiting, and difficulty in swallowing.

F

False Bittersweet (American Bittersweet) – can cause vomiting and diarrhea.

False Hellebore – is toxic if eaten, and may cause nausea and vomiting.

False Queen Anne's Lace – leads to photosensitization resulting to ulcerative and exudative dermatitis

Feather Geranium – can cause vomiting, anorexia, and depression.

Fern Palm – can cause vomiting (may be bloody), dark stools, jaundice, increased thirst, bloody diarrhea, bruising, liver failure, death. One to two seeds can be fatal.

Fetterbush – can cause vomiting, diarrhea, weakness, and cardiac failure.

Fiddle-Leaf – can cause oral irritation, intense burning and irritation of mouth, tongue, and lips, excessive drooling, vomiting, and difficulty in swallowing.

Fig – may lead to gastrointestinal and dermal irritation.

Figwort – can cause vomiting, diarrhea, depression, anorexia, hypersalivation, and wobbly gait.

Fire Lily – can cause vomiting, salvation, diarrhea; large ingestions cause convulsions, low blood pressure, tremors, and cardiac arrhythmias. Bulbs are the most poisonous part of this plant.

Flag – can cause salivation, vomiting, drooling, lethargy, and diarrhea. Highest concentration is in rhizomes.

Flamingo Flower – can cause oral irritation, pain and swelling of mouth, tongue, and lips, excessive drooling, vomiting, and difficulty in swallowing.

Florida Beauty – Vomiting (occasionally with blood), depression, anorexia, hypersalivation.

Florist's Calla – Oral irritation, intense burning and irritation of mouth, tongue and lips, excessive drooling, vomiting, and difficulty in swallowing.

Foxglove – can cause cardiac arrhythmias, vomiting, diarrhea, weakness, cardiac failure, and may lead to death.

Franciscan Rain Tree – can cause tremors, seizures for several days, diarrhea, vomiting, hypersalivation, lethargy, loss of coordination, and coughing.

G

Garden Chamomile – may lead to contact dermatitis, vomiting, diarrhea, anorexia, and allergic reactions. Long-term use can lead to bleeding tendencies.

Garden Hyacinth – can cause vomiting, diarrhea, dermatitis, and allergic reactions. Bulbs contain highest amount of toxin.

Gardenia – may result in mild vomiting and/or diarrhea and hives.

Garlic – can cause vomiting, breakdown of red blood cells (hemolytic anemia, Heinz body anemia), blood in urine, weakness, high heart rate, and panting.

Gaultheria – is harmful if eaten in quantity.

Geranium – can cause vomiting, anorexia, depression, and dermatitis.

Geranium Leaf Aralia – may lead to contact dermatitis, vomiting, anorexia, and depression.

Giant Dracaena – can cause vomiting (occasionally with blood), depression, anorexia, and hypersalivation.

Giant Dumb Cane – can cause oral irritation, intense burning and irritation of mouth, tongue, and lips, excessive drooling, vomiting, and difficulty in swallowing.

Giant Hogweed – may result in photosensitization (ulcerative and exudative dermatitis) and ocular toxicity.

Glacier Ivy – can cause vomiting, abdominal pain, hypersalivation, and diarrhea. Foliage is more toxic than berries.

Gladiola – can cause salivation, vomiting, drooling, lethargy, and diarrhea. Highest concentration is in corms (bulbs).

Gloriosa Lily – may cause salivation, vomiting (bloody), diarrhea (bloody), shock, kidney failure, liver damage, and bone marrow suppression.

Gold Dieffenbachia – can cause oral irritation, pain and swelling of mouth, tongue, and lips, excessive drooling, vomiting, and difficulty in swallowing.

Gold Dust Dracaena – can cause vomiting, depression, inappetence, drooling, incoordination, and weakness.

Golden Birds nest – can cause nausea, vomiting, and diarrhea.

Golden Pothos – can cause oral irritation, intense burning and irritation of mouth, tongue, and lips, excessive drooling, vomiting, and difficulty in swallowing.

Golden Ragwort – may lead to liver disease if ingested in large amount or over a long time period.

Good Luck Plant – All parts of the plant have toxic potential, although the possibility of serious effects is usually limited to ingestions of large quantities. Consuming *oxalis* species can produce kidney failure if significant amounts are eaten.

Grapefruit – can cause vomiting, diarrhea, depression, and may lead to potential dermatitis. Fruit is edible. The skins and plant material can cause problems.

Grass Palm – can cause vomiting (occasionally with blood), depression, anorexia, and hypersalivation.

Greater Ammi – can cause oral irritation, intense burning and irritation of mouth, tongue and lips, excessive drooling, vomiting, and difficulty in swallowing.

Green Gold Naphthysis – can cause oral irritation, intense burning and irritation of mouth, tongue and lips, excessive drooling, vomiting, and difficulty in swallowing.

Ground Apple – can cause contact dermatitis, vomiting, diarrhea, anorexia, allergic reactions. Long-term use can lead to bleeding tendencies.

Grundsel – The plant is not very palatable but will be eaten by animals with no other forage; poisonings typically occur from ingestion of green plant material or material in hay. The toxic components can cause liver failure, which is referred to as *walking disease* or *sleepy staggers*. Signs of poisoning include weight loss, weakness, sleepiness, yawning, incoordination, yellowish discoloration to mucous membranes (*icterus*), neurologic problems secondary to liver failure (aimless walking, chewing motions, head pressing). Animals may appear to be normal at first, then become suddenly affected; the syndrome progresses rapidly over a few days to a week. Liver damage, depression, anorexia, vomiting, diarrhea, muddy mucous membranes, weakness, and ataxia are some of its possible results.

H

Hahn's Self Branching Ivy – may result in vomiting, abdominal pain, hypersalivation, and diarrhea. Foliage is more toxic than berries.

Hashish – may result in prolonged depression, vomiting, un-coordination, sleepiness or excitation, hypersalivation, dilated pupils, low blood pressure, low body temperature, seizure, coma, and death.

Hawaiian Ti – may result in vomiting (occasionally with blood), depression, anorexia, and hypersalivation.

Heartleaf Philodendron – can cause oral irritation, pain and swelling of mouth, tongue, and lips, excessive drooling, vomiting, and difficulty in swallowing.

Heavenly Bamboo – may result in weakness, un-coordination, seizures, coma, respiratory failure, and death.

Hellebore – can cause drooling, abdominal pain and diarrhea, colic, and depression.

Hercules' Club – may result in skin and oral irritation, hypersalivation, vomiting, and diarrhea.

Hills of Snow – may result in vomiting, depression, and diarrhea. Cyanide intoxication is rare and usually produces more of a gastrointestinal disturbance.

Holly – can cause vomiting, diarrhea, and depression. Leaves and berries are low in toxicity.

Hops – may result in panting, high body temperature, seizures, and death.

Horse Chestnut (Buckeye) – may result in severe vomiting and diarrhea, depression or excitement, dilated pupils, coma, convulsions, and wobbly.

Horsehead Philodendron – can cause oral irritation, intense burning, and irritation of mouth, tongue, and lips, excessive drooling, vomiting, and difficulty in swallowing.

Horseweed – may result in mild vomiting and diarrhea.

Hortensia – may result in vomiting, depression, diarrhea. Cyanide intoxication is rare and usually produces more of a gastrointestinal disturbance.

Hosta – can cause vomiting, diarrhea, and depression.

House Pine – may lead to vomiting and depression.

Hurricane Plant – causes oral irritation, intense burning and irritation of mouth, tongue, and lips, excessive drooling, vomiting, and difficulty in swallowing.

Hyacinth – can cause intense vomiting, diarrhea (occasionally with blood), depression, and tremors.

Hydrangea – may result in vomiting, depression, and diarrhea. Cyanide intoxication is rare and usually produces more of a gastrointestinal disturbance.

I

Impala Lily – may result in vomiting, diarrhea, anorexia, depression, irregular heartbeat, and death.

Indian Apple – can cause vomiting, diarrhea, lethargy, panting, coma (rare); dermal may result in redness and skin ulcers.

Indian Borage – causes vomiting, diarrhea, depression, anorexia, occasionally bloody diarrhea or vomiting.

Indian Hemp – may result in diarrhea (possibly with blood), slow heart rate, and weakness.

Indian Pink – causes depression, diarrhea, vomiting, excessive salivation, abdominal pain, and heart rhythm disturbances.

Indian Rubber Plant –

Inkberry – can cause vomiting, diarrhea and depression. Leaves and berries are low in toxicity.

Iris – may result in salivation, vomiting, drooling, lethargy, diarrhea, Highest concentration is in rhizomes.

Iron Cross Begonia – causes kidney failure, vomiting, and salivation in dogs. Most toxic part is underground.

Ivy Arum – can cause oral irritation, intense burning and irritation of mouth, tongue, and lips, excessive drooling, vomiting, and difficulty in swallowing.

J

Jack-in-the-pulpit – may result in oral irritation, pain and swelling of mouth, tongue, and lips, excessive drooling, vomiting (not horses), and difficulty in swallowing.

Jade Plant – causes vomiting, depression, and un-coordination.

Japanese Yew – may result in tremors, difficulty breathing, vomiting, seizures, and sudden death from acute heart failure. Early signs include muscular tremors and dyspnea.

Jerusalem Cherry – leads to gastrointestinal disturbances, possible ulceration of the gastrointestinal system, seizures, depression, respiratory depression, and shock.

Jerusalem Oak – causes vomiting, anorexia, and depression.

Jonquil – leads to vomiting, salvation, and diarrhea; large ingestions cause convulsions, low blood pressure, tremors and cardiac arrhythmias. Bulbs are the most poisonous part.

K

Kaffir Lily – may result in vomiting, salvation, diarrhea; large ingestions cause convulsions, low blood pressure, tremors and cardiac arrhythmias. Bulbs are the most poisonous part.
Kalanchoe – causes vomiting, diarrhea, and abnormal heart rhythm.
Kiss-me-quick – leads to tremors, seizures (for several days), diarrhea, vomiting, hypersalivation, lethargy, incoordination, and coughing.
Klamath Weed – may result in photosensitization (ulcerative and exudative dermatitis).
Kudu lily – causes vomiting, diarrhea, anorexia, depression, irregular heartbeat, and may lead to death.

L

Lace Fern – may result in allergic dermatitis with repeated dermal exposure. Berry ingestion could result in gastric upset (vomiting, abdominal pain, or diarrhea.)
Lace Tree Philodendron – causes oral irritation, pain and swelling of mouth, tongue, and lips, excessive drooling, vomiting, and difficulty in swallowing.
Lady-of-the-night – leads to tremors, seizures (for several days), diarrhea, vomiting, hypersalivation, lethargy, incoordination, and coughing.
Lambkill – can cause vomiting, diarrhea, weakness, and cardiac failure.
Lantana – causes vomiting, diarrhea, labored breathing, weakness, and liver failure.

Larkspur – The toxicity of the plant may vary depending on seasonal changes and field conditions; as the plant matures, it generally becomes less toxic. The alkaloids in the plant cause neuromuscular paralysis; clinical effects include constipation, colic, increased salivation, muscle tremors, stiffness, weakness, recumbence, and convulsions. Cardiac failure may occur, and can lead to death from respiratory paralysis.

Laural – causes vomiting, diarrhea, weakness, and cardiac failure.

Lavender – leads to nausea, vomiting, and inappetence.

Leatherflower – may result in salivation, vomiting, and diarrhea.

Leak – causes vomiting, breakdown of red blood cells (hemolytic anemia, Heinz body anemia), blood in urine, weakness, high heart rate, and panting.

Lemon – may result in vomiting, diarrhea, depression, and potential dermatitis. Fruit is edible while skins and plant material can cause problems.

Lemon Grass – causes stomach upset, difficulty breathing, weakness, and may lead to death.

Lemon Verbena – causes stomach upset and colic. No concerns if small amounts are used in cooking or as flavoring agent.

Lemon Rose – may result in drooling, abdominal pain and diarrhea, colic, and depression.

Lily-of-the-palace – causes vomiting, salvation, diarrhea; large ingestions cause convulsions, low blood pressure, tremors, and cardiac arrhythmias. Bulbs are the most poisonous part.

Lily-of-the-valley – may result in vomiting, irregular heartbeat, low blood pressure, disorientation, coma, and seizures.

Lily-of-the-valley Bush – causes vomiting, diarrhea, depression, cardiovascular collapse, hypersalivation, weakness, coma, low blood pressure, and death. Ingestion of a few leaves can cause serious problems.

Lime – may lead to vomiting, diarrhea, depression; potential dermatitis. Fruit is edible while skins and plant material can cause problems.

Lobelia – causes depression, diarrhea, vomiting, excessive salivation, abdominal pain, and heart rhythm disturbances.

Locust – causes vomiting, depression, anorexia, weakness, difficulty breathing, diarrhea (bloody), and death.

Lord-and-Ladies – causes oral irritation, intense burning and irritation of mouth, tongue and lips, excessive drooling, vomiting, and difficulty in swallowing.

Lovage – causes diuretic and increased urination.

M

Macadamia Nut – may lead to depression, weakness (especially of rear limbs), vomiting, and tremors.

Madagascar Dragon Tree – may result in vomiting (occasionally with blood), depression, anorexia, and hypersalivation.

Maidens Breath – causes vomiting and diarrhea.

Malanga – leads to oral irritation, intense burning and irritation of mouth, tongue, and lips, excessive drooling, vomiting, and difficulty in swallowing.

Maleberry – can cause vomiting, diarrhea, depression, cardiovascular collapse, hypersalivation, weakness, coma, low blood pressure, and death. Ingestion of a few leaves can cause serious problems.

Mapleleaf Begonia – causes kidney failure, vomiting, and salivation. Most toxic part is underground.

Marble Queen – Symptoms of poisoning are intense burning of the mouth, throat, and lips, and difficulty in breathing.

Marijuana – may result in prolonged depression, vomiting, incoordination, sleepiness or excitation, hypersalivation, dilated pupils, low blood pressure, low body temperature, seizure, coma, and death.

Marjoram – causes vomiting and diarrhea.

Mauna Loa Peace Lily – may lead to oral irritation, pain and swelling of mouth, tongue and lips, excessive drooling, vomiting (not horses), and difficulty swallowing.

Mayapple – can cause vomiting, diarrhea, lethargy, panting, coma (rare); dermal leads to redness and skin ulcers.

Mayweed – leads to contact dermatitis, vomiting, diarrhea, anorexia, and allergic reactions. Long-term use can lead to bleeding tendencies.

Meadow Saffron – causes oral irritation, bloody vomiting, diarrhea, shock, multi-organ damage, and bone marrow suppression.

Medicine Plant – may cause vomiting and change in urine color to red

Metallic Leaf Begonia – may result in kidney failure, vomiting, and salivation. Most toxic part is underground.

Mexican Breadfruit – causes oral irritation, intense burning and irritation of mouth, tongue, and lips, excessive drooling, vomiting, and difficulty in swallowing.

Milfoil – leads to vomiting, diarrhea, depression, anorexia, and hypersalivation.

Milkweed – causes vomiting, profound depression, weakness, anorexia, and diarrhea are common; it may be followed by seizures, difficulty in breathing, rapid, weak pulse, dilated pupils, kidney or liver failure, coma, respiratory, paralysis, and death.

Mint – can cause vomiting and diarrhea with large ingestions.

Mistletoe – causes vomiting, diarrhea, low blood pressure (rare), difficulty in breathing, and low heart rate.

Mock Azalea – causes vomiting, diarrhea, anorexia, depression, irregular heartbeat, and death.

Mole Bean Plant – Access to ornamental plants or pruned foliage is most common in poisonings. Ricin is a highly toxic component that inhibits protein synthesis; ingestion of as little as one ounce of seeds can be lethal. Signs typically develop from twelve to forty-eight hours after ingestion. Symptoms include loss of appetite, excessive thirst, weakness, colic, trembling, sweating, loss of coordination, difficulty in breathing, progressive central nervous system depression, and fever. As syndrome progresses, bloody diarrhea may occur, and convulsions and coma can precede death.

Morning Glory – causes vomiting and large amounts of seeds may cause hallucinations.

Morning-noon-and-night – may result in tremors, seizures (for several days), diarrhea, vomiting, hypersalivation, lethargy, incoordination, and coughing.

Moss Rose – causes kidney failure, tremors, and salivation.

Mother of Millions – may result in vomiting, diarrhea, and abnormal heart rhythm.

Mother-in-Law – causes oral irritation, intense burning, and irritation of the mouth, lips, and tongue, excessive drooling, vomiting, and difficulty in swallowing.

Mother-in-Law Plant – may lead to vomiting, diarrhea, and abnormal heart rhythm.

Mother-in-Law's Tongue – causes nausea, vomiting, and diarrhea.

Mum – may result in vomiting, diarrhea, hypersalivation, incoordination, and dermatitis.

N

Naked Lady – may lead to vomiting (not horses), depression, diarrhea, abdominal pain, hypersalivation, anorexia, and tremors.

Nandina – causes weakness, incoordination, seizures, coma, respiratory failure, and death.

Narcissus – may cause vomiting, salvation, and diarrhea; large ingestions cause convulsions, low blood pressure, tremors and cardiac arrhythmias. Bulbs are the most poisonous part.

Nasturtium (Watercress) – causes mild vomiting and diarrhea.

Needlepoint Ivy – may lead to vomiting, abdominal pain, hypersalivation, and diarrhea. Foliage is more toxic than berries.

Nephthytis – causes oral irritation, pain and swelling of mouth, tongue, and lips, excessive drooling, vomiting, and difficulty in swallowing.

Nicotiana (Tobacco) – leads to hyper-excitability then depression, vomiting, incoordination, paralysis, and death is possible.

Nightshade – may lead to hypersalivation, inappetence, severe gastrointestinal upset, diarrhea, drowsiness, CNS depression, confusion, behavioral change, weakness, dilated pupils, and slow heart rate.

Norfolk Island Pine – causes vomiting and depression.

O

Octopus Tree – causes mild vomiting, diarrhea.

Oilcloth Flower – may lead to oral irritation, intense burning and irritation of mouth, tongue, and lips, excessive drooling, vomiting, and difficulty in swallowing.

Oleander – causes drooling, abdominal pain, diarrhea, colic, depression, and death.

Onion – may lead to vomiting, breakdown of red blood cells (hemolytic anemia, Heinz body anemia), blood in urine, weakness, high heart rate, and panting.

Orange – causes vomiting, diarrhea, depression, and potential dermatitis. Fruit is edible, skins and plant material can cause problems.

Oregano – may lead to mild vomiting and diarrhea.

Oregon Holly – causes vomiting, diarrhea, and depression. Leaves and berries are low toxicity.

Ornamental Pepper – may lead to gastrointestinal disturbances, possible ulceration of the gastrointestinal system, seizures, depression, respiratory depression, and shock.

P

Pacific Yew – can cause tremors, difficulty breathing, vomiting, seizures (dogs), and sudden death from acute heart failure.

Painter's Pallette – may lead to oral irritation, intense burning and irritation of mouth, tongue, and lips, excessive drooling, vomiting, and difficulty in swallowing.

Palm Lily – causes vomiting (occasionally with blood), depression, anorexia, and hypersalivation.

Panda Plant – may cause to oral irritation, intense burning and irritation of mouth, tongue, and lips, excessive drooling, vomiting, and difficulty in swallowing.

Paper White – leads to vomiting, salvation, and diarrhea; large ingestions cause convulsions, low blood pressure, tremors and cardiac arrhythmias. Bulbs are the most poisonous part.

Paraguayan Jasmine – may lead to tremors, seizures (for several days), diarrhea, vomiting, hypersalivation, lethargy, incoordination, and coughing.

Parsley – may result in photosensitization leading to sunburn and dermatitis; large amounts are needed to cause this effect.

Peace Begonia – causes kidney failure, vomiting, and salivation. Most toxic part is underground.

Peace Lily – may lead to oral irritation, intense burning and irritation of mouth, tongue, and lips, excessive drooling, vomiting, and difficulty in swallowing.

Peach – Stems, leaves, seeds contain cyanide, and particularly toxic in the process of wilting, which can result in brick red mucous membranes, dilated pupils, difficulty breathing, panting, and shock.

Peacock Flower – causes vomiting and diarrhea.

Pencil Cactus – is irritating to the mouth and stomach, and sometimes causes vomiting.

Peony – causes vomiting, diarrhea, and depression.

Perennial Pea – leads to weakness, lethargy, pacing, head pressing, tremors, seizures, and possible death.

Periwinkle – may lead to vomiting, diarrhea, low blood pressure, depression, tremors, seizures, coma, and death.

Philodendron Pertusum – causes oral irritation, pain and swelling of mouth, tongue, and lips, excessive drooling, vomiting (not horses), and difficulty in swallowing.

Pie Plant – leads to kidney failure, vomiting, and salivation. Most toxic parts are leaves and roots.

Pieris – may cause vomiting, diarrhea, depression, cardiovascular collapse, hypersalivation, weakness, coma, low blood pressure, cardiovascular collapse, and death. Ingestion of a few leaves can cause serious problems.

Pig Lily – causes oral irritation, intense burning and irritation of mouth, tongue, and lips, excessive drooling, vomiting, and difficulty in swallowing.

Pigtail Plant – leads to oral irritation, intense burning and irritation of mouth, tongue, and lips, excessive drooling, vomiting, and difficulty in swallowing.

Pink Pearl – causes kidney failure, tremors, and salivation.

Pinks – may lead to mild gastrointestinal signs and mild dermatitis.

Plantain Lily – can cause vomiting, diarrhea, and depression.

Plum – Stems, leaves, and seeds contain cyanide, and particularly toxic in the process of wilting, which may cause brick red mucous membranes, dilated pupils, difficulty breathing, panting, and shock.

Plumosa Fern – leads to allergic dermatitis with repeated dermal exposure. Berry ingestion could result in gastric upset (vomiting, abdominal pain, or diarrhea.)

Poinciana – causes intense burning and irritation of mouth, tongue and lips, excessive drooling, vomiting, diarrhea, difficulty in swallowing, and lack of coordination.

Poinsettia – can be irritating to the mouth and stomach, and can sometimes cause vomiting.

Poison Daisy – may lead to contact dermatitis, vomiting, diarrhea, anorexia, and allergic reactions. Long-term use can lead to bleeding tendencies.

Poison Hemlock – leads to agitation, tremors, drooling, diarrhea, paralysis, and death.

Poison Parsnip – can cause diarrhea, seizures, tremors, extreme stomach pain, dilated pupils, fever, bloat, respiratory depression, and death.

Portulaca – causes muscle weakness, depression, and diarrhea.

Pothos – may lead to oral irritation, intense burning and irritation of mouth, tongue, and lips, excessive drooling, vomiting, and difficulty in swallowing.

Prayer Bean – leads to severe vomiting and diarrhea (sometimes bloody), tremors, high heart rate, fever, shock, and death. Seeds are very toxic (seed coat must be broken).

Precatory Bean – may lead to severe vomiting and diarrhea (sometimes bloody), tremors, high heart rate, fever, shock, and death. Seeds are very toxic (seed coat must be broken).

Pride-of-India – causes diarrhea, vomiting, salivation, depression, weakness, and seizures. Ripe fruit/berries are most toxic but the bark, leaves, and flowers are toxic too.

Primrose – can cause mild vomiting.

Privet – may lead to gastrointestinal upset (most common), incoordination, increased heart rate, and death.

Purlane – leads to muscle weakness, depression, and diarrhea.

Q

Queensland Nut – can cause depression, weakness (especially of rear limbs), vomiting, and tremors to dogs.

R

Racemose asparagus – causes allergic dermatitis with repeated dermal exposure. Berry ingestion could result in gastric upset (vomiting, abdominal pain, or diarrhea).

Ragwort – The plant is not very palatable, but it will be eaten by animals with no other forage; poisonings typically occur from ingestion of green plant material or material in hay. The toxic components can cause liver failure, referred to as *walking disease* or *sleepy staggers*. Signs of poisoning include weight loss, weakness, sleepiness, yawning, incoordination, yellowish discoloration to mucous membranes (*icterus*), neurologic problems secondary to liver failure (aimless walking, chewing motions, and head pressing). Animals may appear to be normal at first, then become suddenly affected; the syndrome progresses rapidly over a few days to a week. It can further cause liver damage, depression, anorexia, vomiting, diarrhea, muddy mucous membranes, weakness, and ataxia.

Ranger's Button – may lead to photosensitization leading to sunburn and dermatitis; large amounts are needed to cause this effect.

Red Emerald – causes oral irritation, intense burning and irritation of mouth, tongue, and lips, excessive drooling, vomiting, and difficulty in swallowing.

Red Princess – causes oral irritation, intense burning and irritation of mouth, tongue, and lips, excessive drooling, vomiting, and difficulty in swallowing.

Red-Marginated Dracaena – may lead to abdominal pain, increased heart rate, drooling, vomiting, depression, inappetence, incoordination, and weakness.

Rex Begonia – causes kidney failure, vomiting, and salivation. Most toxic part is underground.

Rhododendron – leads to vomiting, diarrhea, hypersalivation, weakness, coma, hypotension, CNS depression, cardiovascular collapse and death. Ingestion of a few leaves can cause serious problems. The toxic principle interferes with normal skeletal muscle, cardiac muscle, and nerve function. Clinical effects typically occur within a few hours after ingestion and can include acute digestive upset, excessive drooling, loss of appetite, frequent bowel movements/diarrhea, colic, depression, weakness, loss of coordination, stupor, leg paralysis, weak heart rate, and recumbency for two or more days;

at this point, improvement may be seen or the animal may become comatose and eventually die.

Rhubarb – causes kidney failure, tremors, and salivation.

Ribbon Plant – may lead to vomiting (occasionally with blood), depression, anorexia, and hypersalivation.

Ridderstjerne – may lead to vomiting, salvation, and diarrhea; large ingestions cause convulsions, low blood pressure, tremors and cardiac arrhythmias. Bulbs are the most poisonous part.

Rock Moss – Symptoms of poisoning are weakness, lethargy, hypersalivation, and tremors leading to kidney failure and death.

Roman Chamomile – leads to contact dermatitis, vomiting, diarrhea, anorexia, and allergic reactions. Long-term use can lead to bleeding tendencies.

Rose of China – causes vomiting, diarrhea, nausea, and anorexia.

Rose of Sharon – causes vomiting, diarrhea, nausea, and anorexia.

Rosebay – causes vomiting, diarrhea, hypersalivation, weakness, coma, hypotension, CNS depression, cardiovascular collapse, and death. Ingestion of a few leaves can cause serious problems. Rhododendron is typically not very palatable to horses unless it is the only forage available, but sheep and goats may graze readily on the plant. The toxic principle interferes with normal skeletal muscle, cardiac muscle, and nerve function. Clinical effects typically occur within a few hours after ingestion and can include acute digestive upset, excessive drooling, loss of appetite, frequent bowel movements/diarrhea, colic, depression, weakness, loss of coordination, stupor, leg paralysis, weak heart rate, and recumbency for two or more days; at this point, improvement may be seen or the animal may become comatose and die.

Running Myrtle – causes vomiting, diarrhea, low blood pressure, depression, tremors, seizures, coma, and death.

S

Sabi Star – causes vomiting, diarrhea, anorexia, depression, irregular heartbeat, and death.

Sacred Bamboo – can cause weakness, incoordination, seizures, coma, respiratory failure, and death.

Saddle Leaf – may lead to oral irritation, intense burning and irritation of mouth.

Sago Palm – The Sago Palm is an extremely poisonous plant to dogs when ingested, causing bloody vomiting and diarrhea, bleeding disorders, liver failure and death.

Satin Pothos – causes oral irritation, pain and swelling of mouth, tongue, and lips, excessive drooling, vomiting, and difficulty in swallowing.

Scented Geranium – results primarily to gastrointestinal upset, and could also cause ataxia, muscle weakness, depression or hypothermia in larger exposures.

Schefflera – may lead to oral irritation, intense burning and irritation of the mouth, lips, tongue, excessive drooling, vomiting, and difficulty in swallowing.

Seaside Daisy – causes mild vomiting and diarrhea.

Seven Bark – leads to vomiting, depression, and diarrhea. Cyanide intoxication is rare, and usually produces more of a gastrointestinal disturbance.

Shamrock Plant – results in kidney failure, tremors, and salivation.

Shatavari – may lead to allergic dermatitis with repeated dermal exposure. Berry ingestion could result in gastric upset (vomiting, abdominal pain, or diarrhea).

Showy Daisy – may lead to mild vomiting and diarrhea.

Silver Dollar – causes nausea and retching.

Silver Jade Plant – causes nausea and retching.

Skunk Cabbage – leads to oral irritation, pain and swelling of mouth, tongue, and lips, excessive drooling, vomiting (not horses), and difficulty in swallowing.

Snake Lily – may result in salivation, vomiting, drooling, lethargy, and diarrhea. Highest concentration is in rhizomes.

Snake Plant – causes nausea, vomiting, and diarrhea.

Solomon's Lily – may lead to oral irritation, intense burning and irritation of mouth, tongue, and lips, excessive drooling, vomiting, and difficulty in swallowing.

Sorrel – leads to small exposures only resulting in gastrointestinal upset. Very large amounts can cause weakness, muscle fasciculation, and potentially seizures from hypocalcemia. Hypocalcemia can also result in arrhythmias. Secondary renal injury may also develop from the crystals; this is only expected in massive exposures or with chronic ingestion.

Sowbread – results in salivation, vomiting, and diarrhea. Following large ingestions of tubers will lead to heart rhythm abnormalities, seizures, and death.

Spanish Thyme (Essential oil) – causes vomiting, diarrhea, depression, anorexia, occasionally bloody diarrhea or vomiting.

Spindle Tree – leads to vomiting, diarrhea, abdominal pain, and weakness. Heart rhythm abnormalities may result from large doses.

Split Leaf Philodendron – causes oral irritation, intense burning and irritation of mouth, tongue, and lips, excessive drooling, vomiting, and difficulty in swallowing.

Spotted Dumb Cane – leads to oral irritation, intense burning and irritation of mouth, tongue, and lips, excessive drooling, vomiting, difficulty in swallowing.

Sprengeri Fern – may lead to allergic dermatitis with repeated dermal exposure. Berry ingestion could result in gastric upset (vomiting, abdominal pain, or diarrhea).

Spring Parsley – may lead to photosensitization resulting to sunburn and dermatitis.

St. John's Wort – may lead to photosensitization resulting to ulcerative and exudative dermatitis.

Staggerbush – causes vomiting, diarrhea, depression, cardiovascular collapse, hypersalivation, weakness, coma, low blood pressure, and death. Ingestion of a few leaves can cause serious problems.

Starch Root – causes oral irritation, intense burning and irritation of mouth, tongue, and lips, excessive drooling, vomiting, and difficulty in swallowing.

Starleaf – While this plant does contain potentially toxic substances, the most common effects seen are mild vomiting and diarrhea.

Stinking Chamomile – may lead to contact dermatitis, vomiting, diarrhea, anorexia, and allergic reactions. Long-term use can lead to bleeding tendencies.

Straight-Margined Dracaena – can cause vomiting, depression, inappetence, drooling, incoordination, and weakness.

Striped Dracaena – can cause vomiting, depression, inappetence, drooling, incoordination, and weakness.

Superb Lily – may lead to salivation, vomiting (bloody), diarrhea (bloody), shock, kidney failure, liver damage, and bone marrow suppression.

Sweet Cherry – Stems, leaves, ands seeds contain cyanide, and particularly toxic in the process of wilting, which leads to brick red mucous membranes, dilated pupils, difficulty in breathing, panting, and shock.

Sweet Pea – causes weakness, lethargy, pacing, head pressing, tremors, seizures, and possible death.

Sweet William – leads to mild gastrointestinal signs and mild dermatitis.

Sweetheart Ivy – causes vomiting, abdominal pain, hypersalivation, and diarrhea. Foliage is more toxic than berries.

Swiss Cheese Plant – leads to oral irritation, intense burning and irritation of mouth, tongue and lips, excessive drooling, vomiting, and difficulty in swallowing.

T

Tahitian Bridal Veil – can cause mild gastrointestinal signs and dermatitis.

Tail Flower – may lead to oral irritation, intense burning and irritation of mouth, tongue, and lips, excessive drooling, vomiting, and difficulty in swallowing.

Taro – causes oral irritation, intense burning and irritation of the mouth, lips, tongue, excessive drooling, vomiting, and difficulty in swallowing.

Taro Vine – causes oral irritation, intense burning and irritation of mouth, tongue and lips, excessive drooling, vomiting, and difficulty in swallowing.

Tarragon (essential Oil) – causes mild vomiting and diarrhea.

Texas Umbrella Tree – leads to diarrhea, vomiting, salivation, depression, weakness, and seizures. Ripe fruit/berries are most toxic but also bark, leaves, and flowers.

Ti (Plant) – causes vomiting (occasionally with blood), depression, anorexia, and hypersalivation.

Tobacco – may lead to hyper-excitability then depression, vomiting, incoordination, paralysis, and possible death.

Tomato Plant – may lead to hypersalivation, inappetence, severe gastrointestinal upset, depression, weakness, dilated pupils, and slow heart rate; ripe fruit is nontoxic.

Tree Philodendron – causes oral irritation, intense burning, and irritation of the mouth, lips, tongue, excessive drooling, vomiting, and difficulty in swallowing.

Tree Tobacco – leads to hyper-excitability then depression, vomiting, incoordination, paralysis, and possible death.

Tropic Snow – leads to oral irritation, intense burning, and irritation of mouth, tongue, and lips, excessive drooling, vomiting, and difficulty in swallowing.

True Aloe – causes vomiting and change in urine color to red.

Trumpet Lily – may lead to oral irritation, intense burning and irritation of mouth, tongue, and lips, excessive drooling, vomiting, and difficulty in swallowing.

Tulip – causes vomiting, depression, diarrhea, and hypersalivation. Highest concentration of toxin is in the bulb.

U

Umbrella Leaf – causes vomiting, diarrhea, lethargy, panting, coma (rare); dermal leads to redness and skin ulcers.

V

Variable Dieffenbachia – may lead to oral irritation, intense burning and irritation of the mouth, lips, tongue, excessive drooling, vomiting, and difficulty in swallowing.

Variegated Philodendron – may lead to oral irritation, intense burning and irritation of the mouth, lips, tongue, excessive drooling, vomiting, and difficulty in swallowing.

Vinca – causes vomiting, diarrhea, low blood pressure, depression, tremors, seizures, coma, and death.

Virgin's Bower – causes salivation, vomiting, and diarrhea.

W

Wahoo – may lead to vomiting, diarrhea, abdominal pain, and weakness. Heart rhythm abnormalities may result from large doses.

Wake Robin – causes oral irritation, intense burning and irritation of mouth, tongue, and lips, excessive drooling, vomiting, and difficulty in swallowing.

Wandering Jew – leads to dermatitis.

Warneckei Dracaena – may lead to vomiting (occasionally with blood), depression, anorexia, and hypersalivation.

Water Flag – causes salivation, vomiting, drooling, lethargy, diarrhea. Highest concentration is in rhizomes (underground stem).

Water Hemlock – leads to diarrhea, seizures, tremors, extreme stomach pain, dilated pupils, fever, bloat, respiratory depression, and death.

Wax Leaf – may result in gastrointestinal upset (most common), incoordination, increased heart rate, and death.

Weeping Fig – Symptoms of poisoning include abdominal pain, agitation, diarrhea, drooling, loss of appetite, mouth pain, skin inflammation, and vomiting.

Western Yew – leads to tremors, difficulty breathing, vomiting, seizures, and sudden death from acute heart failure.

White Heads – may result in photosensitization leading to ulcerative and exudative dermatitis, and ocular toxicity.

Wild Arum – causes oral irritation, intense burning and irritation of mouth, tongue, and lips, excessive drooling, vomiting, and difficulty in swallowing.

Wild Calla – causes oral irritation, intense burning and irritation of mouth, tongue, and lips, excessive drooling, vomiting, and difficulty in swallowing.

Wild Carnation – leads to mild gastrointestinal signs and mild dermatitis.

Wild Coffee – may lead to contact dermatitis, vomiting, anorexia, and depression.

Winter Cherry – may lead to gastrointestinal disturbances, possible ulceration of the gastrointestinal system, seizures, depression, respiratory depression, and shock.

Winterberry – causes vomiting, diarrhea, and depression. Leaves and berries are low in toxicity.

Wisteria – causes vomiting (sometimes with blood), diarrhea, and depression.

Y

Yarrow – leads to increased urination, vomiting, diarrhea, and dermatitis.

Yellow Oleander – causes vomiting, diarrhea, and slow heart rate.

Yesterday, Today, Tomorrow – may lead to tremors, seizures (for several days), diarrhea, vomiting, hypersalivation, lethargy, incoordination, and coughing.

Yew – may result in sudden death from acute cardiac failure; early signs are muscular tremors, dyspnea, and seizures in dogs.

Yew Pine – causes severe vomiting and diarrhea.

Yucca – causes vomiting.

Essential Plant Oils

Some plant oils and essential oils have been known to cause seizures in dogs although there are some good essential oils that are identified in the chapter on "Holistic Treatments of Seizures". Listed below are the essential oils to avoid:

- Camphor
- Eucalyptus
- Fennel
- Hyssop
- Pennyroyal

Rosemary

- Sage
- Savin
- Spanish thyme
- Tansy
- Tarragon
- Tea tree
- Thuja
- Turpinetine
- Wormwood

Chapter 22

What is the Immune System?

The immune system is a defensive mechanism of organs and cells designed to protect the dogs' body against invading pathogens like parasites, toxins, viruses, fungi, bacteria, infectious diseases, and cancers. A well-balanced immune system reduces the risk of these diseases and contributes to the overall health of your dog. The components of the immune system are the skin, the gastrointestinal tract, the lungs, the mucosal lining of surface areas of the body, and most importantly, the blood. These parts of the immune system identify harmful pathogens coming into the body, and then work to eliminate the threat.

The other important role of the immune system is to ensure that the cells are functioning properly. If they are old, cancerous, or just malfunctioning, the immune system works to remove these cells.

There are two types of immune responses

When a parasite, infection, virus, or bacteria tries to invade the dog's body, the immune system has two responses that occur together in unison to fight the invader. These are the specific immunity and the nonspecific immunity.

1. **Specific Immunity or Adaptive Immune System**

After the body has been exposed to a foreign pathogen, the specific immunity gets to work to eliminate the invader or prevent it from growing. It learns about the substance, remembers it, adapts to it, and is able to respond to that pathogen the next time it attacks. This way, the specific immune system can prevent a reoccurrence of certain pathogens.

When your dog gets an immunization vaccine shot, the veterinarian is deliberately introducing an immune response from the immune lymphocytes B-cells and T-cells produced by stem cells in the bone marrow. The B-cells respond with antibodies containing proteins called immunoglobulin. The antibodies in the white blood cells travel though the body looking for foreign pathogen and binds to it to make it inactive.

2. **Nonspecific or Innate Immune System**

The cells in this immune system, by way of white cells, recognize and respond to pathogens similarly to the specific immune system but does not provide long lasting protection but an immediate defense instead. It sends immune cells to the infected site and identify and remove the foreign pathogen.

Under Active Immune System (Immunodeficiency)

When the dog's body is too weak to fight infectious diseases, cancer, toxins, and other pathogens, the result is an under active immune system. This can be hereditary caused by mutations in the cells, or by viral infections, poor nutrition, insufficient calorie intake, lack of vitamins and minerals, use of steroids, vaccinations, or an extensive injury. Diseases such as parvo, distemper, diabetes, lupus, and renal failure can also lower the immune system. Other factors of immunodeficiency are advanced age, poor nutrition, toxic environment, immunosuppressant drugs (steroids), and genet

Over Active Immune System (Autoimmune)

When the body's immune system attacks itself, this is called autoimmune or over active immune. This is caused by the malfunction of the white blood cells and can cause canine lupus, Addison's disease, psoriasis, rheumatoid arthritis, allergies and others. The exact cause is unclear, but genetic changes can be one of the reasons including other factors such as toxins, stress, or infections. Others suggest possible causes are unnecessary vaccines, food preservatives, excessive use of antibiotics, and chemicals found in pesticides. Symptoms in dogs are diarrhea, anemia, joint pain, weakness, lack of appetite, lethargy, skin lesions, and seizures. Treatment for autoimmune steroids may be administered by a veterinarian, but prolonged use of steroids can cause kidney or liver dysfunction.

Nutrition and the Immune System

Nutrition is the most important factor in keeping a strong, functioning, healthy immune system. Poor nutrition can increase infections, slow down the healing process, and increase susceptibility to disease—the most common cause of immunodeficiency.

A mineral or vitamin deficiency has an important influence on immune response. A deficiency in any nutrient can weaken an immune system, Give your dog nutrients from food rather than supplemental vitamins and minerals, because food nutrients are absorbed faster and better than supplements. Most supplements have less than a 40 percent absorption rate. Amino acid has been linked to increased T-cell function in the immune system and t-cells directly attack foreign pathogens, infections, virus, bacteria, and cancers. Foods high in amino acids (arginine) are flax seed, chicken, salmon, eggs, and soy beans.

Your dog must be eating foods rich in antioxidants bolsters the immune system. Antioxidants protect cells from oxidation that damages cells and slow the aging process. Carotenoids are foods that contain antioxidants. They are the fruits and vegetables that are red, orange, and yellow in color.

Lycopene is a carotenoid found in tomatoes (red vegetable) while lutein is a carotenoid found in corn (yellow vegetable). If you're not sure if your dog is getting enough antioxidants in his diet, especially from a commercial dog food, a good supplement would help to ensure your dog has a healthy immune system and protection from toxins and pathogens.

Fresh food contains live bacteria (the good kind), and unfortunately dry commercial dog food has none. Consider a probiotic supplement for your dog. It's generally safe and the extra beneficial bacteria helps in the digestive system and the immune system.

The Gastrointestinal Tract and the Immune System

The gastrointestinal tract is of primary importance when it comes to the immune system. The gastrointestinal tract contains approximately 60 percent of the entire immune system, compared to any other organ. This is where most of pathogens enter the body, along with the nutrients needed, so the immune system has to be very selective in what is absorbed and what is excreted from a dog's body. Some things can support the immune system and some can damage it.

Stress and the Immune System

Stress is the body's reaction to any stimuli that disturbs its natural order, and if that stress is chronic, it has a negative effect on the immune system. Stress or anxiety plays a large role in the health of your dog. It affects the dog's behavior, emotional well-being, the heart, skin, and the whole immune system. Some of the things that cause dogs stress are:

- boredom,
- lack of exercise,
- poor diet,
- poor living conditions,
- fighting in the home, and lack of attention.

Thyroid Disease and the Immune System

Autoimmune Thyroiditis (Hypothyroidism)

This is an autoimmune disorder where the immune cells of the body are attacking the thyroid gland. The thyroid compensates by producing more of the hormone thyroxine until the gland is depleted of the hormone. Canine hypothyroidism is a condition in which the thyroid cannot produce enough of the hormone thyroxine for the body.

Thyroxine is a hormone that maintains the metabolic rate, body temperature, and regulates growth and development. Another reason the thyroid cannot produce enough hormone is the thyroid will shrink with age and will produce less and less. Dogs that are genetically predisposed to this disorder are; Airedale terriers, boxers, cocker spaniels, dachshunds, Doberman pinschers, golden retrievers, greyhounds, Irish setters, Labrador retrievers, and miniature schnauzers. Symptoms are weight gain, hair loss, dry skin, chronic infections of the ear or skin, slow heart rate, dull dry coat, and behavior change including seizures. Treatment is shot of a synthetic hormone thyroxine that must be continued for the rest of the dog's life.

Hyperthyroidism

Hyperthyroidism is an overactive thyroid that produces too much thyroxine. This condition is rare compared to hypothyroidism. If a dog has hypothyroidism and is given too much medication or a high dosage of synthetic thyroxine, the symptoms are the same as an overactive thyroid gland. Symptoms are rapid breathing, dull coat, restlessness, Irritability and hyperactivity. Treatment can involve surgery but the dog will have to take medication for the rest of its life.

Treatment of Immune Disorders

Treatment for Over Active Immune System (Autoimmune)

The treatment of autoimmune disease will be done with immune suppressing drugs that will hold back the hyperactivity of the immune system. The veterinarian will consider prescribing a corticosteroid such as prednisone, prednisolone, or dexamethasone. These drugs are steroids and have many side effects both short term and long-term including liver and kidney failure. Because the drugs basically reduce or shut down the immune system, it leaves the dog vulnerable and the treatment needs to be closely supervised by a veterinarian. There are other considerations in using natural remedies to bring back a balance to the immune system using plant sterols or steroilins. Adding fatty acids, digestive enzymes, and probiotics to ensure the digestive tract has a balance of good bacteria that will fight the incoming bad bacteria. The dog should be in a stress free environment since stress destroys the immune system. Adding antioxidants to the body as in coenzyme Q10 will help reduce the free radicals in the body.

Treatment for Under Active Immune System (Immunodeficiency)

Under active immune systems happen usually in the case of after an illness, over vaccination, old age, use of steroid drugs, protein malnutrition, insufficient caloric intake, insufficient vitamins or minerals, disease or stress. Illnesses like diabetes, renal failure, and lupus can lower the immune system. There are many treatments like immune enhancing drugs that can be given to the dog including antibiotics. For an under active immune system, there are many nutrients you can give your dog. Start with multiple vitamins and minerals: B complex (good for stress) and Vitamins A, C, and E. Minerals like selenium has a high amount of antioxidants and zinc. Some herbs are a good immune booster for an underactive immune system: suma, cats claw, burdock, echinacea, goldenseal, red clover, and dandelion. It's important that the dog gets fresh food in its diet for good nutrition rather than dry dog food—at least until the dogs has gain its heath back.

CHAPTER 23

Yard and Garden

A. Insecticides

Areas which are prone to flea and tick infestations tend to use various forms of insecticide: e.g., organophosphates and carbamates. But exposure to insecticides, especially after heavy applications of chemicals, are toxic to dogs. Dogs exposed to toxic chemicals may not exhibit all of the signs of poisoning. In fact, sometimes insecticides will cause the opposite of these symptoms instead, but there will usually be some indication that the dog is not well. If you suspect that your dog is unwell because of exposure to insecticides, you will need to remove your dog from the toxic environment or cease using the insecticides, and seek medical attention before the condition becomes dire. The symptoms of insecticide poisoning are as follows: fever, vomiting diarrhea, anorexia, depression, muscle tremors, hypersalivation, constricted pupils, increased heart rate, lack of coordination, seizures, and respiratory failure.

Carbamate – Toxic levels of carbamate insecticides like methomyl and carbofuran can cause seizures and respiratory arrest in your dog. Signs of carbamate toxicity in dogs include: vomiting, diarrhea, drooling, breathing problems, muscle tremors, twitching, weakness, and paralysis. Veterinary care is required immediately, and bathing the dog to remove the toxin from the skin. If ingested, an active charcoal solution should be administered by your veterinarian. Some of the carbamate toxins are:

Aldicarb – an active ingredient in Temik, and is ffective against aphids and spider mites.

Carbaryl – an active ingredient in Sevin and targets mosquitoes.

Carbofuran – is the most toxic carbamate pesticides. It is marketed under the trade names Furadan, by FMC Corporation and Curater, among several others.

Fenoxycarb – is used for fire ant, fleas, mosquitoes, and cockroach control. It has a low toxicity to dogs.

Methiocarb – is used as snail bait and is highly toxic to dogs. Hyperthermia (overheating due to tremors and seizures) – is a major complication. Treatment includes supportive care (intravenous fluids, often anesthesia, oxygen, and potentially mechanical ventilation) administered by a veterinarian.

Methomyl – is highly toxic to dogs and is used to control spiders and ticks. It is readily absorbed through the skin or the lungs.

Oxamyl – is highly toxic to dogs. Used to control mites and ticks. Can enter the body by inhalation, ingestion, and skin absorption.

Propoxur – is used in flea collars. Quickly absorbed.

Thiodicarb – is registered to be used on sweet corn only. It has a low risk when it comes to dogs. It can be ingested though the skin or lungs.

Organophosphate – its toxicity may lead to chronic anorexia, muscle weakness, and muscle twitching which may last for days or even weeks. Dogs will seek out organophosphate products when mixed with tasty fertilizers and bone meal. Organophosphate insecticides inhibit cholinesterases and acetylcholinesterase, which are essential enzymes in the body. Cholinesterases are enzymes which break down acetylcholine, a neurotransmitter. Consequently, acetylcholine remains attached to the postsynaptic receptors of the neurons causing continuous and unending nervous transmission to nervous tissue, organs, and muscles (smooth and skeletal). This causes seizures and shaking. Some organophosphate lawn and garden insecticides commonly used include:

Acephate – is used to control aphids, fire ants, caterpillars, and other insects. Dogs that ate acephate granules had vomiting, diarrhea, shaking, and difficulty walking and breathing.

Chlorpyrifos – is used in dog flea collars, flea sprays, and dog shampoos as well as termite and cockroach pesticide. Since it is a neurotoxin it can cause dizziness, increased urination, salivation, seizures, and death.

Coumaphos – symptoms include vomiting, diarrhea, anorexia, depression, hypersalivation, increased heart rate, respiratory failure, and seizures.

Cyothioate – as a tablet, it is ingested by dogs to control flea infestation. This insecticide has low effects on dogs if administered correctly.

Diazinon – can be absorbed through the skin, and has been reported to cause acute pancreatitis in dogs. Symptoms include trouble breathing, diarrhea, uncontrolled twitching, seizures, and death.

Dimethoate – this is not as toxic as others but can be inhaled or absorbed in the skin and in sufficient doses can cause death.

Disulfoton – can be inhaled, ingested, or absorbed through the skin, and can cause increased heart rate, and pancreatitis.

Fampfhur – may lead to vomiting, diarrhea, depression, muscle tremors, hypersalivation, increased heart rate, seizures, and respiratory failure.

Fention – can cause vomiting, diarrhea, depression, muscle tremors, hypersalivation, increased heart rate, seizures, and respiratory failure.

Fonofos – can be inhaled, ingested, or absorbed through the skin. Symptoms include fever, vomiting, diarrhea, anorexia, depression, muscle tremors, hypersalivation, increased heart rate, seizures, and respiratory failure.

Malathion – can be inhaled, ingested, or absorbed through the skin. Symptoms include fever, vomiting, diarrhea, anorexia, depression, muscle tremors, hypersalivation, increased heart rate, seizures, and respiratory failure.

Parathion – can be inhaled, ingested, or absorbed through the skin. It can also cause liver damage. Symptoms include fever, vomiting, diarrhea, anorexia, depression, muscle tremors, hypersalivation, increased heart rate, seizures, and respiratory failure.

Phosmet – can be found in some dog collars. Symptoms include fever, vomiting, diarrhea, anorexia, depression, muscle tremors, hypersalivation, increased heart rate, seizures, and respiratory failure.

Ronnel – is used in cattle. Symptoms include fever, vomiting, diarrhea, anorexia, depression, muscle tremors, hypersalivation, increased heart rate, seizures, and respiratory failure.

Terbufos – is used on corn and grain, and is extremely toxic for dogs. Symptoms include fever, vomiting, diarrhea, anorexia, depression, muscle tremors, hypersalivation, increased heart rate, seizures, and respiratory failure.

Tetrachlorvinphos – is found in flea and tick spray and collars. Symptoms include fever, vomiting, diarrhea, anorexia, depression, muscle tremors, hypersalivation, increased heart rate, seizures, and respiratory failure.

Trichlorfon – can be inhaled, ingested, or absorbed through the skin. Symptoms may include vomiting, diarrhea, anorexia, depression, muscle tremors, hypersalivation, increased heart rate, seizures, and respiratory failure.

Other toxic insecticides are:

Abamectin – is a bait used to control cockroaches and plant parasites. It is also known as nematicide. Symptoms include eye and skin irritation, vomiting, convulsions, seizures, tremors, and respiratory failure.

Amitraz – is known as a *monoamine oxidase inhibitor (MAOI)*. Common side effects of the insecticide include sedation and dry skin. Serious side effects include low blood pressure, decreased body temperature, elevation of blood glucose, dilated pupils, slow heart rate, slowed intestinal rate, *ataxia*, prolonged sedation, vomiting, diarrhea, and seizures. Death may occur.

Bifenthrin – Bifenthrin is also an insecticide in the Pyrethroid family. Pyrethroids are manmade versions of pyrethrins, which come from chrysanthemum flowers. Products containing bifenthrin come in many forms, including sprays, granules, and aerosols. Symptoms include fever, vomiting, diarrhea, anorexia, depression, muscle tremors, hypersalivation, increased heart rate, seizures, and respiratory failure.

Permethrin – is a synthetic insecticide in the Pyrethroid family, and is found in many types of flea and tick control products. The most common signs are tremors, drooling, lack of appetite, vomiting, diarrhea, incoordination, hyperactivity, disorientation, vocalization, depression, difficulty breathing, and seizures. Death may occur.

Dogs who come into contact with lawn pesticides may encounter several health issues including seizures. Moreover, pesticides may trigger seizures in dogs who already have epilepsy. Besides seizures, dogs may become lethargic, develop glandular issues, suffer from liver and kidney problems, and exhibit other indications of toxicity. In many instances, the canine may die from exposure or over exposure to lawn chemicals. If you suspect that your dog is unwell because of exposure to insecticides, you will need to remove your dog from the toxic environment or cease using the insecticides, and seek medical attention from a veterinarian for it before the condition becomes dire. It is crucial that you provide information about any insecticides you think your dog has been exposed to, including those used on your lawn, in your garden, and on your pet.

Below is a list of insecticides that, when used as directed, can be safer to use around pets:

- Acetamiprid
- Imidacloprid
- Lufenuron
- Nitenpyram
- Pyriproxyfen
- S-Methoprene
- Spinosad

Dogs are closer to the surface than humans are. They place their noses on the ground, in the grass, into bushes and shrubs, and plants and flowers. Dogs are very nosy. Moreover, canines walk with unprotected feet. The pesticide and herbicide residue attaches itself to the paws. Dogs, as is their nature, lick their paws. They also lick other parts of the body exposed to the toxic chemicals. As a result, they ingest the poisonous materials.

Never apply outdoor insecticides while your pet, any toys, or feeding bowls, are on the lawn. Avoid pellet pesticides that can be mistaken for food. When storing insecticides, make sure they are out of reach and locked up so that children and animals cannot access them. Don't mix insecticides with organic fertilizer—most dogs like the taste of organic fertilizers. When your pet is outside, it can be harder to protect them from dangerous insecticides. Your neighbor's pesticides can also drift into your lawn and affect your pet. It is best to get to know your neighbor and talk to them about their pesticide use so that you know which pesticides to stay away from, since it is advisable avoid treated areas for at least seventy-two hours and waiting longer is better. If you suspect your dog or cat has been poisoned by an insecticide, contact an emergency veterinarian and poison control immediately. It's important to gather as much information as possible:

- What is the poisonous chemical around the yard or may have been available?
- How much was ingested?
- What is the means of exposure?

Bring the insecticide packaging if you can; if your pet has <u>vomited</u>, bring a small vomit sample for analysis. Depending on how long it has been since your pet ingested the toxin (if exposure was via ingestion), your veterinarian may induce vomiting for your pet. Your doctor may also wash out your pet's stomach with a tube (lavage), and then give it activated charcoal to detoxify and neutralize any remaining insecticide. Antidotal treatments specific to the toxin will also be given to your pet. Further treatment may include an oxygen cage if your pet is having trouble breathing, and fluid therapy if your pet has been unable to drink or is <u>anorexic</u>.

Prevention

Treatment is possible but, as so many dog owners have found, it is futile. After immediate or ongoing exposure to pesticides, many dogs die. They suffer needless beforehand before passing. A proactive approach is best. Do not use any form of commercial and chemical pesticide or herbicide on your lawn or garden. Make sure your neighbors are aware of your stance. This will, hopefully, prevent their provider from spraying onto your property. Make sure the lawn company posts signs with the name of the product clearly indicated. This will help in case of exposure. If an incident happens, hold the company responsible. If possible, contact the city council or appropriate body for a pesticide ban.

To treat your own lawn, turn to animal and environmentally friendly products. Check online for these alternatives. Talk to a garden store and other sources for possible information. If you do have to use harsh chemicals, take all the necessary precautions. Spray according to the directions. Keep your pet in a well-ventilated area, away from the spraying. Wash the paws immediately upon coming back inside.

Conclusion

The spraying of chemicals on the lawn is an accepted practice by many individuals. Yet, more evidence is surfacing to question the safety of the use of chemicals. It seems they are harmful to the water, the air, people, and, even moreso, pets. Increasingly, many individuals are turning to natural solutions. In some states and cities, pesticide and herbicide use is banned.

B. Herbicides

How are the dogs being exposed to these toxic chemicals?

They can directly ingest these chemicals from sprayed lawns and weeds or they can lick their paws and fur where the chemicals were picked up. There are guidelines for the application of herbicides, but can you be sure that your neighbor has read and followed the directions on the packaging?

Some common herbicides—specifically 2,4 (dichlorophenoxyacetic acid, 2,4-D), 4-chloro-2-methylphenoxypropionic acid (MCPP), and dicamba — remained detectable on grass for at least forty-eight hours after application, and the chemicals persisted even longer on grass under certain environmental conditions. These chemicals can be tracked inside the house and contaminate flooring and furniture. Dog owners may come in contact with the chemicals simply by petting or holding their pets during walks. Roundup and similar herbicides are not as dangerous as disulfoton and snail bait, but they can still cause <u>vomiting</u> if eaten. Put your dogs inside along with their <u>chew toys, food bowls</u>, and anything else they might put their mouths when applying herbicides, and make sure they stay there until the treated area is good and dry. Once it's dry, the chemical has been taken down to the root of the plant, and the lawn is considered dog-safe.

To avoid dog exposure to herbicides, homeowners should always store, mix, and dilute products in areas that pet do not have access. Gastrointestinal upset is the most common sign seen when ingestion of fertilizer and herbicide occurs, and if large amounts or concentrated products are ingested, veterinary intervention may be necessary. Dogs whose owners use a herbicide containing 2,4-D are up to twice as likely to develop lymphatic cancer—a finding that suggests that the plant–killing chemical may be a health risk to humans.

You might also try using corn gluten meal in place of chemicals: a natural herbicide, it's effective and safe for dogs.

List of Herbicides.

Atrazine – is a herbicide of the trazine class, and is used to prevent broad leaf weeds on lawns. OSHA studies determined that the toxicity is low for dogs in low doses. In high doses, the symptoms are vomiting, shaking, and convulsions.

Benefin – is for broad leaf weeds and crab grass control, and is irritating to the eyes and skin.

Bensulide – is a selective organophosphate herbicide, is used on vegetable crops to control annual grasses, and can trigger seizures, dogs may become lethargic, development of glandular issues, and sufferring from liver and kidney problems.

Dacthal (DCPA) – is used as a herbicide for broad leaf in lawns, and it contains dioxin, a low level toxin, but its long-term exposure will have adverse effects on the liver, adrenal gland, kidneys, thyroid, and spleen.

Dicamba – is a benzoic acid herbicide used to control broadleaf plants, brush, and vines. It can be inhaled, ingested, or absorbed through the skin. Symptoms are skin irritation, eye irritation, congested lungs, and inflamed kidneys.

DSMA – is an arsenical compound containing cacodylic acid and is cancer causing (carcinogen). Symptoms are vomiting, diarrhea, muscle weakness, hypothermia, lethargy, seizures, and death.

Endothall– Symptoms of poisoning are vomiting, diarrhea, damaged intestinal walls, and hemorrhages in the stomach.

Glyphosate – Symptoms of poisoning are skin irritation, vomiting, diarrhea, damaged to liver, and pancreas.

MCPA– is a 4-chloro-2-methylphenoxyacetic acid used as a herbicide in the
   control of annual and perennial weeds. Symptoms are diarrhea, jaundice, loss of weight, lethargy and anemia.

MCPP – 4-chloro-2-methylphenoxypropionic acid (MCPP/Mecoprop) and is associated with high risk of bladder cancer in dogs. Symptoms are lethargy, liver and kidney problems, seizures, and death.

Siduron – is used for crab grass control. Symptoms are vomiting, diarrhea, muscle tremors, increased heart rate, lack of coordination, and trouble breathing.

MSMA – is used for weed control, and can be inhaled, ingested, or absorbed through the skin. Symptoms are lethargy, liver and kidney problems, seizures, and death.

Oxadiazon – is used for roadside weed control. Symptoms are vomiting, diarrhea, muscle tremors, increased heart rate, lack of coordination, and trouble breathing.

Pronamide – It can be inhaled, ingested, or absorbed through the skin. Symptoms are vomiting, diarrhea, muscle tremors, increased heart rate, lack of coordination, and trouble breathing.

C. Rodenticides, Avicides, Predacides, Mollusicides

Rodenticides

Bromethalin – is a toxic substance that is found in a variety of rat and mice poisons. Ingestion can lead to an increased pressure of cerebrospinal fluid (the liquid within the membrane of the skull that the brain essentially floats in) and cerebral edema (the accumulation of excess water in the brain). A variety of neurological-based symptoms can result from this, including muscle tremors, seizures, and impaired movement.

Strychine – is a rat poison can be inhaled, ingested, or absorbed through the skin; it is very painful. Symptoms include violent seizures, muscle stiffness, increased heart rate, respiratory failure, and death.

Thallium – is a rat poison. Symptoms include vomiting, severe abdominal pain, diarrhea, trembling, and death.

Zinc phosphate – can turn into phosphine—a toxic gas in the stomach. It is used as rat bait. Symptoms include vomiting, anxiety, stagger, or loss of coordination.

Any dog who has been exposed to a rodenticide should receive immediate attention from a veterinarian.

Avicides

4-Aminopyridine – is known by the trade name Avitrol and is mainly used to control birds (avicide). Symptoms include dizziness, breathing difficulty, tremors, salivation, and seizures.

Predacide

Sodium Flouroacetate – is a highly toxic predacide used to control foxes, wild dogs, coyotes, and feral pigs. Mixed with meat bait domestic dogs would easily be lured to these baits. Signs include anxiety, vomiting, shaking, frenzied behavior, seizures, convulsions and death.

Molluscicide

Metaldehyde – is used as a snail and slug bait. Symptoms include muscle tremors, anxiety, hyperesthesia, ataxia, hyperthermia, diarrhea, and seizures.

Slug and snail bait with metaldehyde.

It can cause tremors, seizures, and even death and again, and it tastes mighty good to dogs. If you have a dog, use something else. Baits containing ferric phosphate are a less toxic version.

D. Toads

Toad venom toxicity is relatively common in dogs. Being natural predators, it is common for dogs to catch toads in their mouths, thereby coming into contact with the toad's toxin, which the toad releases when it feels threatened. This highly toxic defense chemical is most often absorbed through the oral cavity membrane, but it may also enter the eyes, causing vision problems. Its effects are lethal if not treated immediately.

The two most important species of toad that are known for their toxic effects on pets are the Colorado River toad and the marine toad. Symptoms usually appear within a few seconds of the toad encounter and may include the following:

- Crying or other vocalization
- Pawing at the mouth and/or eyes
- Profuse drooling of saliva from the mouth
- Change in the color of membranes of the mouth – may be inflamed or pale
- Difficulty in breathing
- Unsteady movements
- Seizures
- High temperature
- Heart abnormalities

E. Fertilizer

Most fertilizers contain varying amounts of nitrogen, phosphorus and potassium (potash) as indicated by the three numbers on the packaging (i.e., 30-10-10). They may also contain iron, copper, zinc, cobalt, boron, manganese, and molybdenum, some of which may be toxic in large concentrations. Additionally, fertilizers may also contain herbicides, pesticides, and fungicides which increases the risk of poisoning. Surprisingly, the more dangerous types of fertilizers are organic fertilizers. Most pet owners want to use safer products around their pets, and so they often reach for something organic. Organic fertilizers are typically natural fertilizers that are leftover byproducts from the meatpacking or farming industry. Examples of these include: bone meal, blood meal, feather meal, and fish meal. Symptoms include drooling, vomiting, severe lethargy, diarrhea, excessive tearing, urinating, abnormal heart rate, difficult breathing, tremors, seizures and death.

F. Bee & Wasp Stings

Bee and Wasp venom – Every dog will react differently when it is stung by a bee or wasp. Some dogs have a little discomfort and will simply howl and itch for a short period, while others could have a severe reaction that could be deadly. The dog's curious nature causes them to get stung mostly on the nose, on the head and in the mouth. If you see your dog get bitten by a bee, your first job is to locate and remove the stinger with your fingernails. If your dog is allergic to bee or wasp stings, the most severe reaction will be to have difficulty breathing, start trembling, have diarrhea, start vomiting and possibly faint. These are all symptoms of your dog experiencing anaphylactic shock and if left untreated can kill your dog in under fifteen minutes. This is why quick observation of his reactions and contact with a doctor are vital early on, it could save your dog's life. Your veterinarian will be able to administer treatment to help with the dog's pain and then keep him overnight for observation.

Chapter 24

Dog Collars

The Collar vs. Harness – Cervical subluxation can also cause seizures, and this is something many pet owners don't realize. This type of seizure occurs alot in dogs that are chained outside. They run out the length of their chain chasing after a neighborhood cat, and when the chain snaps back against the neck, it causes a high cervical traumatic injury of either the C1 vertebrae (the atlas) or C2 (the axis). The C1 is the first cervical vertebrae in animals, and it articulates with the brain stem. When there is increased cerebrospinal fluid pressure in the brain stem, and it can lead to a seizure.

It is recommend you harness your pet not only for walks, but also if he's ever chained out. It's important that your pet is not able to increase pressure on the neck, because <u>high cervical subluxations and other chiropractic issues in the neck</u> can caused an increased likelihood of seizures.

Bark Collars – if a dog is prone to having epilepsy or seizures, sound or vibration from a collar may trigger this seizure.

Shock / Static Collars – Shock is actually using pain to correct the dog and electronic impulses can trigger seizures. Shocking is a more intense correction.

Chapter 25

Stress

Stress in dogs is now recognized as Canine Stress Syndrome or CSS and is known as a hereditary disorder that is characterized by muscle tremors, muscle rigidity and seizures. Stress or anxiety will cause seizures in a dog that already has epilepsy and any stressful event can trigger a seizure. Some of the stress factors/triggers that can bring on a seizure is listed below.

- Changes in routine caused by construction, visitors, new family members, etc.
- Being left alone
- Car rides
- Visits to the vet
- Thunderstorms
- Changes in barometric pressure
- Extreme cold weather
- Flashing lights from TV, cameras, Christmas trees or lightning
- Angry voices
- Loud arguments between people (dogs think you are angry at them and it is the worst kind of stress for them)
- Fatigue
- Nervousness

- Anxiety
- Going too long between meals
- Prolonged excitement
- Any changes, sudden, subtle, radical, etc. (food, environment, etc.)
- Medications

Some of the treatment for dogs prone to stress is to be on a glucose replacement therapy to replace the depleted blood sugar. Another treatment is to put the dog on tranquilizers to reduce the level of stress, especially during the periods of times that the dog is under high stress: i.e., thunderstorms, car rides, angry voices, etc. Also, feeding a dog frequent smaller meals each day is better than one or two larger meals because this helps the dog to maintain his blood sugar levels during the day.

Chapter 26

The Household

Cleaning Products

Many products we use in the home for clean are very toxic to dogs. It is important to store all your cleaning products when not in use. Keep a poison control phone number taped to your cabinet close to your phone in case of an emergency. Any cleaning product with ingredients of ammonia, bleach, chlorine, glycol ethers, or formaldehyde are toxic. Some of the toxic cleaning agents are:

Pine-Sol (or cleaners with pine oil) – The fumes from a pine-sol container can cause burns on the inside of the throat and nose of a dog, and may even severely damage the lungs. After the cleaner is applied to the floor, the vapors will linger and pose a danger to your pet.

- Mister Clean
- Clorox Bathroom Cleaner
- Clorox Toilet Bowl Cleaner
- Scrubbing Bubbles
- Windex
- Formula 409

Scented Candles

Scented Candles contain many toxins. The candle industry is not regulated and labeling is not required. Burning candles in your home reduces the air quality and adds pollution which can contribute to conditions such as asthma and allergies. The smoke from a scented candle burning can release dangerous chemicals into the air such as carcinogens, and neurotoxins, just like cigarette smoke. Some of these toxins are:

Paraffin – a petroleum based chemical that release carcinogens.

Lead – is used as a metal core for the wicks. U.S. candle companies volunteered to stop using lead in their candles but imported candles still use lead in their wicks.

Acrolein, Formaldehyde, Acetaldehyde – all of them are carcinogens.

Benzene – can be inhaled and is a carcinogen.

Toluene – can be inhaled and affects the central nervous system.

Perfume

Perfume, as well as after shave, contains ethanol—a toxin to dogs. Add an essential oil, and you have something that a dog smells 1000 times more than a human that affect them in a bad way.

Pennies

Zinc and lead are the most common culprits. The most common cause of zinc toxicities is ingestion of pennies. Pennies minted since 1983 are primarily zinc and some dogs love to ingest coins. Clinical signs are gastrointestinal upset and anemia from red blood cell destruction. Surgery is usually necessary to remove the pennies to prevent further absorption of zinc. The best treatment is prevention so keep your pocket change in a jar out of your dog's reach.

Carpet Shampoo

Most carpet cleaning products can be used in pet households. The carpet must be allowed to dry before allowing pets into the area. This will help to prevent the risk of skin irritation or gastrointestinal upset.

Carpet Fresheners

Proper use of carpet deodorizing products should not cause significant harm or injury to pets. Should your pet accidentally come in contact with the freshly applied powder, we recommend washing the paws with mild soap and water to avoid minor skin irritation. Minor ingestions of carpet freshener powder generally results in a mild stomach upset. If a small amount is inhaled, minor respiratory irritation may occur, resulting to sneezing, coughing, or a runny nose. Because of this, it is a good idea to continue to keep your dog out of the room until after you have vacuumed up the powder.

Bleach

If your dog has ingested a bleach-containing product or a drain cleaner, do not induce vomiting. As always, contact poison control with the product name and the approximate amount ingested and seek emergency veterinary care. There is always a risk associated with cleaning their pets' cages and toys with bleach. Cleaning your pet's cage or toy with a properly diluted bleach solution and followed by a thorough rinsing and airing out will prevent any harm.

Essential Oils

Dogs are sensitive to essential oils and effects may be gastrointestinal upset, central nervous system depression, and even liver damage could occur if ingested in significant quantities. Inhalation of the oils could lead to aspiration pneumonia. There are significant variations in toxicity among specific oils. Based on this, we would not recommend using essential oils in areas where your pets have access, unless pets are supervised or the use of the oil is approved by your veterinarian.

Fabric Softener Sheets

Fabric softeners contain cationic detergents. These detergents have the potential to cause significant signs like drooling, vomiting, oral and esophageal ulcers, and fever. These clinical signs do require treatment by a veterinarian. Oral ulcers can develop if a pet chews on a new, unused dryer sheet. Used sheets have minimal amounts of detergent. If an animal ingests enough sheets, used or dry, an intestinal blockage may occur.

Loud Music

A dog's hearing is far better than yours or mine. Dogs can hear seven times better than the average human. In fact, your dog may hear something before you do. He may even be hearing something that you are completely unable to hear.

Cigarette Smoke

Pets have a greater risk of passive cigarette smoke then humans because they stay home more, in an environment that has residue of smoke everywhere, furniture, dogs coat, carpet, curtains, etc. Study after study show that dogs who live with smokes have a higher percentage of lung cancer, and nasal tumors and cancer. A dog, (and cat) will groom itself by licking his fur and take in and ingesting anything on its fur including toxic particles for smoking.

Cigarette butts

Cigarette butts contain a high concentrated level of nicotine and other toxins. If a dog ingests a butt it can be fatal. A cigarette butt contains 4 to 8 milligrams of nicotine. Five milligrams of nicotine is fatal to a dog. A toxic level of nicotine is 5 to 1 milligram of nicotine per pound of dog.

Symptoms of nicotine poisoning is constricted pupils, vomiting, diarrhea, fast heartbeat, drooling, twitching, and seizures.

Nicotine Patches and Nicotine gum

A dog will get into garbage or anything laying on the floor and chew it and swallow it. A cigarette patch contains from 8 to 114 milligrams of nicotine.

Dogs can be attracted to nicotine gum because of the sweetness and ingest it. Sometimes the sweetener is xylitol, which is a toxin to dogs. The gum contains about 4 milligrams of nicotine.

E-cigarettes

E-cigarette liquid (known as e-liquid or e-juice) is used to recharge the cartridge for an e-cigarette. The amount of nicotine in these bottles could easily kill a dog if the contents were ingested. Often the liquid is flavored, making the product more appealing. As such, we urge pet parents to keep all tobacco products out of their pets' reach. If accidental ingestion occurs, seek veterinary help immediately.

Breath Fresheners

Human breath mints and breath fresheners are not safe to use on your dog. Certain breath strips contain menthol, which can be irritating to the tissues of the mouth and the gastrointestinal tract.

Some breath-freshening products could also contain the sweetener xylitol, which has the potential to cause a sharp drop in a dog's blood sugar, resulting in depression, loss of coordination, and seizures; in some cases, this could even result in liver damage. If you wish to control your dog's breath problem, we recommend talking with your veterinarian to discuss a safe and appropriate oral hygiene program.

Kaopectate and Pepto Bismol

These products contain salicylates, which are similar to aspirin. Depending on the circumstances of exposure, large enough doses of bismuth salicylate could cause effects similar to aspirin poisoning. These include gastric irritation or ulceration, bleeding problems, seizures, and liver damage.

Mosquito Repellent

Pet owners should never use any product on their animal that is not specifically created for them. Certain mosquito repellents that are made for human beings contain DEET (N, N-diethyl-meta-toluamide). The use of DEET on pets is not recommended, as dogs and cats are very sensitive to it and may develop neurological problems such as tremors, seizures, and death if the product is used on them. If you want to keep mosquitoes away from your dog, we suggest asking your veterinarian for an appropriate product to use.

Batteries

Ingestion of the whole battery as well as chewing on batteries can lead to pain, oral inflammation, hypersalivation, ulceration, vomiting, anorexia, and gastrointestinal upset. Animals may ingest batteries while chewing on other items such as remote controls or battery run toys. X-rays should be taken to see if there are battery parts in the gastrointestinal tract and may require surgery. Seek veterinary attention.

Aspirin, Baby Aspirin

We frequently hear from pet parents who are curious to know if low doses of these medications are safe to use on their pets as a joint and general pain reliever. There are medical conditions where aspirin is a recommended treatment. However, overdosing can result in medical conditions ranging from gastrointestinal upset to liver failure. We strongly advise owners to never give their pets any medication without first consulting with their regular veterinarian. Many drugs, including aspirin, can cause serious or potentially life-threatening problems, depending on the dose involved. If you feel that your dog needs pain relief for any reason, we highly recommend that you get in touch with your veterinarian so that your dog can be evaluated.

Bar Soap and Face Wash

Most bar soaps and face cleansers contain detergents, which, if ingested, can cause gastrointestinal irritation including vomiting and diarrhea. If the soap also contains essential oils such as lavender, for example, it is possible that minor central nervous system depression could occur, depending on the concentration of oils and other circumstances of exposure. Certain soaps are made from glycerin or other emollients, which can have a cathartic effect—causing loose stools or diarrhea. If gastrointestinal signs become persistent, they could lead to dehydration. If a large portion or entire bar of soap were to be ingested, it could potentially lead to obstruction of the animal's gastrointestinal tract. Because of these concerns, we advise keeping your soaps and cleansers in an area that is not accessible to your dog

Toilet Tank Drop Ins/Toilet Water

The drop in products often are made of a corrosive cleaning age. Due to the dilution of the toxin in the toilet tank and bowl, the concentration is usually not very high. Typical clinical sign include gastrointestinal irritation which could include vomiting and diarrhea.

Topical Creams/Ointments

As with lotions and oils, pet parents should use caution after immediate application of topical creams and ointments to their own skin. Always read the label so you know which ingredients are included. Some ingredients found in creams and ointments can cause serious, even life-threatening, clinical signs.

Bread Dough

Ingestion of bread dough can cause gastrointestinal obstruction, vomiting, diarrhea, blindness, inability to walk, vocalization, chance in behaviors and loss of consciousness. Bread dough will rapidly rise in the warm environment of the stomach and produce ethanol. Ethanol is rapidly absorbed from the gastrointestinal tract causing the clinical signs. Prognosis is good if treated immediately by a veterinarian.

Liquid Potpourri

Clinical signs can include skin irritation, oral ulcerations (from grooming or ingestion), corneal erosions and ulcer, irritation of the eye, excessive salivation, vomiting, bloody vomit and diarrhea, and difficult breathing due to inflammation of the upper airway. There may be long-term damage to the esophagus if the materials were ingested causing strictures or perforations. If inhaled, long-term damage to the lungs is also possible. Prognosis depends on what organs and what quantity of agents the pet was exposed to. Decontamination and supportive care is often needed and must be treated by a Veterinarian.

Eucalyptus

Eucalyptus may be hailed for its many benefits, but it should never be consumed by dogs. The effects of eucalyptus ingestion include diarrhea, vomiting, excessive drooling, lethargy, and depression. If you suspect your dog has consumed eucalyptus, or he is presenting with any symptoms attributed to consumption of this toxic plant, immediately consult his veterinarian or an animal poison control hotline.

Camphor

Camphor is generally used in topical pain or arthritis rubs and creams because it is readily absorbed in the skin. Some of the common trade names are Vicks VapoRub, Tiger Balm, Campo-Phenique and Carmex. Campor is poisonous to dogs and should never be used on them. Symptoms of poisoning are skin irritation, nausea, vomiting, diarrhea, depression, and seizures which can lead to death.

Kerosene for lamps

Kerosene (hydrocarbons) is a liquid that is commonly found in your garage. Examples include engine oil, tiki-torch fuels, gasoline, diesel fuels, paint solvents, wood stains, wood strippers, liquid lighter fluids, asphalt/roofing tar, etc. These are often referred to as petroleum distillates based on their viscosity (e.g., thickness), carbon chain length, and fat solubility. Hydrocarbons consist of chemicals containing a hydrogen and carbon group as their main constituents. Some of these products are mixed with <u>antifreeze</u>, which can be deadly to dogs. If your dog or cat ingested hydrocarbons, one should *never* induce vomiting, as it can make the pet worse and predispose them to aspiration pneumonia (e.g., when vomitus is inhaled into the lungs). Clinical signs of hydrocarbon poisoning

include vomiting, drooling, increased breathing, skin irritation, eye irritation, walking drunk, and coma.

Mothballs

Mothballs contain naphthalene and is toxic to dogs. Symptoms include vomiting, diarrhea, increased drinking, urination, and seizures.

PART III

TREATMENTS FOR SEIZURE

Introduction to Part III

Treatments for preventing seizures

The treatments for seizures are usually decided and administered by your veterinarian after a thorough exam and a full range of tests to see if he can determine the cause of the seizures. The fact is, most dog owners never find the cause, and the conventional treatment for the dog is to be put on phenobarbital and/or potassium bromide. This is the beginning of blood tests every six months in order to keep an eye on the liver for damage. The important thing is to look at all the options out there as far as medication and alternative solutions are concerned. Once the dog started the medication, regardless of the chosen solution, the diet must be changed also, because the dog will become less active and lethargic, and he will require a leaner diet.

Each dog reacts differently to the medications given. Your veterinarian may decide to give your dog a combination of medications to find what's right for the dog, and it may take weeks to find out the right amount of dosage and frequency. Medications must be taken every day to be effective and once started must not be discontinued nor skipped or the results could be a severe seizure. Any change must be agreed to by your veterinarian. Other drugs that have been used to treat epilepsy in dogs include felbamate, gabapentin, levetiracetam (keppra), and zonisamide. In general, most dogs on anticonvulsant therapy will need to continue the medication for life. Approximately 20 to 30 percent of dogs cannot be controlled with phenobarbital alone or may become refractory to treatment and start having seizures again.

At this time, a phenobarbital level should be tested to determine if it is at the therapeutic level. Phenobarbital levels should be checked every six months. If the dog is at the maximum therapeutic level of phenobarbital but still having seizures, then potassium bromide or another anticonvulsant may be added. Remember though, that the long-term use of these drugs will contribute to the toxic buildup that can further cause further seizures.

Phenobarbital requires careful monitoring for liver damage and slow increases and decreases in dosages to prevent toxicity and withdrawal symptoms. Some dogs respond better to primidone—a barbituate that metabolizes to phenobarbitol in the dog's body.

There are alternatives to medications and drugs as shown in this part of the book and for the sake of the dog with seizures, It might be the treatment that will work for your dog. If a treatment fails, there are many reasons why; the most common is the owner's lack of administering the medication or improper diagnosis. See a veterinarian neurologist if control is not achieved within three months or if the diagnosis is uncertain.

CHAPTER 27

Seizure Medications

For seizures, most dogs can be controlled by using phenobarbital or phenobarbital and potassium bromide. Potassium bromide is used alone if the dog's liver has become damaged by phenobarbital. Both phenobarbital and potassium bromide are available by prescription in pill, capsule, and liquid form. If your dog does not gain control of seizures with the use of phenobarbital and/or bromide, your vet may refer you to a neurologist who may prescribe one of the other drugs listed here. Most of these medications have an adverse effect on the liver or kidneys if there is prolonged use. Note the side effects of the medication you use, to determine if there is any reaction, and notify the vet. Concentrations of the medication in the blood stream must be monitored in order to control the side effects. Every medication has a time (life) in the body where it is effective, then it is eliminated from the body through metabolism or excretion. Thus, medications like phenobarbital have a half-life of thirty-six to seventy-two hours and others have a half-life of two hours. There is an amount of time that the medication needs to get into the blood stream and get up to an optimum level to begin working. This can be as much as two weeks before a steady state is reached.

Phenobarbital (PB)

Phenobarbital is an anticonvulsant used to control seizures and epilepsy in dogs. It's the most widely used prescription medication used to treat seizures in dogs. This drug controls the number of and severity of seizures in a dog. It works by decreasing the neuron activity in the brain, the glutamate neurotransmitters and increasing the GABA or the gamma-aminobutyric acid in the neurotransmitter to reduce activity level of the neuron. Veterinarians prescribe phenobarbital in tablet or liquid form based on your dog's weight. It is most effective when given twice a day at twelve-hour intervals, and takes ten to fifteen days to have a steady concentration in the body. Phenobarbital reacts with certain other drugs, including anticoagulants, antihistamines, diazepam, phenytoin sodium, corticosteroids, opiate agonists, phenothiazine, doxycycline, furosemide, rifampin, quinidine, metronidazole, theophylline, and valproic acid. Your veterinarian needs to know if your dog is being treated with any other medication prior to begin treatment with Phenobarbital.

Phenobarbital is relatively inexpensive, easy to use and is effective in most seizure cases.

Dosage – The usual dosage to treat seizures is 1 to 1.8 mg per pound every twelve hours, but that depends on the severity of seizures and the dog's weight. The dosage can be increased to 8 mg per pound of body weight if the dog is not responding to the lower dosage.

Side Effects – With the decrease of the neurotransmitters in the brain from the drug, common side effects are lethargy, weakness in the hind legs, loss of coordination, increased appetite, anemia, anxiety, increased thirst, and increase in urination. One of the more serious side effects are the scarring of the liver and liver failure. It is very important to have your veterinarian monitor the liver function when placing your dog on phenobarbital. This should be done every two weeks.

Decreasing or stopping the use of Phenobarbital

The veterinarian will decide on how much to reduce the dosage or eliminate the Phenobarbital medication based blood levels, seizures, side effects and the vets experience in controlling seizures. Decrease the phenobarbital dose is done, once the phenobarbital level reaches 25 mg/dL. This usually takes about one month of treatment. If there are no seizures after six months of therapy, decreasing the phenobarbital is warranted. Note that if you change the dose of phenobarbital it takes about ten to fourteen days for the blood level to equalize at the new level. If the dog has minimal side effects, decreasing the phenobarbital by about 20 percent, and wait a month or two to monitor for seizures. If there are none, then repeat. In some cases, it is desirable to decrease the phenobarbital faster. An example would include a dog with substantial side effects like wobbly gait, lethargy, or liver failure. Frequent monitoring of blood levels during withdrawal is very helpful in these cases.

Potassium Bromide (KBr)

Potassium bromide is an anticonversant used to control seizure by itself or along with phenobarbital. The combination of the two drugs have shown to control seizures in about 70 to 80 percent of dogs. The dog who starts a treatment with potassium bromide has a timeline of four months of dosage before the drug is at the effective level of treatment. For some dogs who have severe seizures, the veterinarian may decide to prescribe a loaded dose of drugs to provide a great sedation of the dog. The dog must be monitored closely to ensure the proper level is maintained and check for side effects. Potassium bromide is considered one of the safest anticonvulsant medications available and it produces fewer side effects than phenobarbital. For that reason, potassium bromide is paired up with phenobarbital to decrease the effects on the liver and reducing the amount of phenobarbital dosage.

Dosage – The starting dosage for potassium bromide is between 13.6 to 18.1 milligrams to a pound of weight. The dosage will be adjusted by your veterinarian based on your dog's reaction to the drug. Dosages come in capsule and liquid form. The liquid form of medication is less expensive, and it's easier to adjust the dosage if that is required. Medication should always be given with food to avoid irritation of the gastrointestinal tract. If the dosage is too high, the dog will have symptoms of in coordination, tremors, lethargy, and paralysis of the hind legs. The dog will require three to four months of treatment for the drug to be fully effective, depending on the absorption rate of potassium bromide, and the metabolism of the dog. Your veterinarian will make adjustments to the dosage on the seizure activity, blood levels, and side effects of the drug.

Side effects of potassium bromide – Side effects include loss of appetite, nausea, thirst, increased urination, sedation, and behavioral changes. Less common side effects in dogs include diarrhea, vomiting, constipation, and pancreatitis. Side effects are more common if the dogs whose potassium bromide concentrations are greater than 2.5 mg/ml but the symptoms usually go away within a week after the dosage is decreased. Some veterinarians switch to sodium bromide, which has all of the anticonvulsant properties, but does not seem to cause gastrointestinal problems.

Decreasing or stopping the use of potassium bromide – sudden discontinue of use of potassium bromide could result in seizures reoccurring in the dog. The dosage must be decreased at a gradual rate over a six month period. Any discontinuing of any medication must be supervised by a veterinarian.

Keppra (Levetiracetam)

Keppra (levetiracetam) is approved in the United States for people with focal seizures refractory to other antiseizure drugs. Since it is a relatively new drug, the optimal dose of levetiracetam (keppra) has not been

determined in dogs. Keppra (levetiracetam) can be used for treating seizures in dogs solely as an anticonvulsant medication. It can also be used in conjunction to phenobarbital and/or potassium bromide. **Keppra is an** *add-on* **drug, and dosage of current antiseizure drugs should be maintained while on keppra. The elimination half-life in dogs is about 3.6 hours. This compares to seven to ten hours in people.**

Dosage – Most neurologists are using 20 mg/kg every eight hours. The veterinarian may alter the dosage depending on the severity of your dog's seizures and adverse side effects to the drug.

Side effects – Keppra has proven to be quite safe for use in dogs with very few side effects. Most dogs seem to tolerate levetiracetam quite well. Side effects which may be seen are drowsiness, changes in behavior and less common effects include gastrointestinal symptoms such as vomiting or diarrhea.

Felbamate

Felbamate (Felbatol) was approved in the United States in 1993 for use in human patients with several types of seizures, including focal seizures. Initial clinical experience indicates that felbamate is often beneficial in dogs with seizures refractory (resistant) to bromide and phenobarbital.

Dosage – A recommended starting dosage is 15 mg/kg. To convert your dog's weight to kilograms, divide the weight by 2.2 every eight hours. The dosage can be increased in 15mg/kg increments every two weeks until seizures are controlled. Dosages as high as 70 mg/kg every eight hours are required and tolerated well in some dogs.

Side effects – Side effects are uncommon although nervousness and hyper-excitability can occur at high doses. Liver disease has been noticed in some dogs taking felbamate in conjunction with phenobarbital, so liver function should be monitored periodically.

The major disadvantages of felbamate are that it is extremely expensive and requires dosing every eight hours.

Primidone

Primidone is similar to phenobarbital but is absorbed into the dogs system at a faster rate after oral administration, with peak levels occurring two to four hours after dosing. primidone is rapidly converted to PEMA (phenylethylmalonamide) and phenobarbital in dogs. All three metabolites PEMA, primidone, and phenobarbital have similar anticonvulsant actions, however primidone is metabolized very rapidly in dogs and contributes very little to the overall antiseizure activity. Phenobarbital, which is metabolized slowly accounts for about 90 percent of the overall antiseizure benefit of the medication. Because primidone is rapidly converted into phenobarbital in dogs, there is some question as to whether it has any advantages over using phenobarbital alone. However, there are a small percentage of dogs who will not respond to phenobarbital, but will respond to primidone. Primadone once commonly used, metabolizes to phenobarbital in the liver.

Dosage – primidone is available in 50 mg and 250 mg tablets and 50 mg/ml suspension. The usual dose for canines is 5 to 15 mg per pound of body weight per day. This is divided into two or three doses to suit individual dog needs. If seizures are not controlled, the dosage might have to be increased. To prevent a relapse, care should be taken to complete the treatment, and avoid sudden discontinuation of the drug. This is advisable even if the dog shows signs of complete recovery. Increasing the dosage might cause severe side effects and decreasing the dosage might increase the chances of the dog suffering a seizure. If a decrease in dosage is recommended, the decrease should be gradual. However, in most cases, the medication has to be administered for life.

Side effects – The disadvantage of primidone is that studies have shown dogs treated with primidone were more likely to show laboratory evidence of liver changes. Based on these factors phenobarbital is generally chosen over primidone as an initial drug to control seizures. With prolonged treatment, it can also cause liver damage.

Gabapentin (Neurontin)

Gabapentin was approved for use in the United States in 1994, and has been used with some success in adult human patients suffering from focal seizures. It is most often used as a secondary/add-on) drug to help treat seizures resistant to phenobarbital and potassium bromide. A major advantage to this drug in humans is that is not metabolized by the liver, so it avoids the hepatoxic (liver injuring) effects of other anticonvulsants. In dogs, gabapentin is metabolized partially by the liver, and no one is completely sure of the anticonvulsant effects of this metabolite. It is believed that gabapentin is beneficial in dogs with focal seizures refractory/resistant to other drugs.

Dosage – A recommended starting dose is 100 to 300 mg per dog given every eight hours. The dose is then adjusted every one to two weeks until seizures are controlled or a maximum dose of 1200 mg every eight hours is reached.

Side effects – The gabapentin's side effects in dogs are limited to mild sedation and ataxia, there are a number of more serious side effects that are associated with exceeding the recommended dosage. When an overdose of gabapentin in dogs occurs the symptoms that would occur include: severe lethargy, sleepiness, somnolence, depression, and intense ataxia. Gabapentin can cause deficiencies in calcium, vitamin D, vitamin B1, and folate. Not only will this make your dog unwell, but because vitamins D and B1 are required for nerve repair, it can also inhibit recovery. Use a multivitamin during treatment to prevent vitamin deficiency. The biggest disadvantages to gabapentin are that it is extremely expensive and requires dosing every eight hours.

Valproic Acid or Valproate (Depakene, Stavzor, Depacon, Depakote)

Valproic Acid is primarily used in combination with other drugs such as phenobarbital. **Valproate (valproic acid) is considered a second line drug for the treatment of epilepsy in dogs.** This medication metabolized very quickly in dogs and therefore its use is limited. **The elimination half-life in dogs is fairly short (approximately three hours). However, these blood levels may still be sufficient in dogs, since lower protein binding of valproate in dogs gives rise to higher brain concentrations, It is used primarily in dogs whose seizures are not well controlled with phenobarbital or bromide; when used in conjunction with other antiseizure drugs, it is mostly phenobarbital or primidone.**

Valproate was successful in reducing seizure frequency by at least 50 percent. Because of the lack of long-term studies and concerns about the rapid metabolism in dogs, its usefulness is in question. **Dosage** – The recommended dosage is 40 to 100 g/ml. The duration of administration of valproic acid depends on the dogs responds to the medication and any adverse side effects.

Side effects – causes nausea and vomiting. These can usually be avoided by giving valproate with or soon after meals. Drowsiness and sedation can occur, especially at higher doses or when valproate is combined with other antiseizure drugs. Hair loss has been observed in dogs.

Diazepam (Valium)

Diazepam is a sedative better known by the brand name valium. The drug is an antianxiety medication and a muscle relaxant for the treatment of epilepsy, seizures, and anxiety. Diazepam increases the production of GABA in the brain which blocks the neurotransmitters that cause dogs to feel excitement. This in turn results in a calm sedative dog in about 30 minutes after dosing.

Dosage – The dosage for diazepam is 0.25mg per pound based on the weight of the dog and is administered every six hours. For dogs having seizures, the medication is usually administered rectally for faster rate of absorption. The veterinarian should always determine the dosage amount for the dog's treatment.
Side effects – Diazepam common side effects are loss of energy, coordinationproblems, slow breathing, and drowsiness. In some cases, the dog may have aggressive behavior, vomiting, anemia, decreased appetite, and liver damage which will show as yellowing eyes, yellowing skin, yellow gums, and depression. An allergic reaction to the drug will show as swelled faces, scratching, hives, pale gums, vomiting, and diarrhea. Some dogs' allergic reaction are seizure and coma. See your veterinarian or emergency animal hospital as soon as possible if these conditions show.

Clorazepate (Tranxene)

Clorazepate was introduced in the United States in 1981. It is sometimes used as add-on treatment for dogs that are unresponsive to first line drugs like phenobarbital or potassium **bromide. After oral administration, clorazepate is converted to nordiazepam (also called N-desmethyldiazepam), in the stomach. Nordiazepam provides all of the antiseizure effect. The elimination half-life is two to five hours, tending to be slightly longer with long-term administration. Sustained release tablets of tranxene offer no pharmacokinetic advantages over regular-release tablets in dogs.**

**Dosage – A dose of 2 mg/kg every eight or twelve hours has been suggested.
Side effects – Co-administration of phenobarbital with clorazepate results in lowered blood levels of clorazepate.**

Tolerance, reduction in antiseizure effects with long-term use can occur with clorazepate, as with most other benzodiazepines.

Lorazepam (Ativan)

Ativan (lorazepam) is prescribed to anxious dogs as an alternative to valium (diazepam). Ativan is part of the benzodiazepine family and has a sedative effect in anxious dogs. It can become physically addictive after periods of prolonged use. **Dosage** – The usual dosage of Ativan for dogs as recommended by vets is 0.02 mg per pound administered once every eight to twelve hours **been suggested.** **Side effect** – Relatively speaking, the drug is quite safe and only begins to present danger at the levels of overdose. Stopping medication suddenly after continuous use extending over a few months is dangerous and can result in side effects such as seizures, vomiting, tremors, cramp, and profuse sweating. Because of this, you will have to slowly taper off the dosage to safely cease use of this medication. Ativan is not given to dogs with liver disease, because it can further damage the liver.

Clonazepam (Klonopin)

Clonazepam is used for maintenance of seizures in dogs. The drug is only effective for a short time requiring frequent administration to maintain adequate serum levels. Also, long-term use of this category of drug reduces its effectiveness in controlling seizures. Long-term use of any benzodiazepine may prevent effective use of to treat emergency seizures. These drugs are effective for the emergency treatment of status epilepsy or cluster seizures. They can also be useful as temporary therapy when seizures can be predicted, such as seizures precipitated by stress or sleep deprivation.

Dosage – The dose range for clonazepam has been reported as 0.05 to 0.25 mg per pound (0.1 to 0.5 mg/kg) orally every eight hours. Your veterinarian will adjust the dosage depending on its effect on your pet, such as signs of excessive sedation, excitement, or poor coordination.

Side effect – While generally safe and effective when prescribed by a veterinarian, clonazepam may cause side effects in some dogs. It should also be avoided in dogs with significant liver disease or glaucoma, and also pregnant dogs because of the risk of birth defects.

Phenytoin (Dilantin)

Although phenytoin is extremely effective in treating human epilepsy, dogs metabolize this drug too quickly to maintain adequate blood levels. More effective antiseizure medications with fewer side effects are available. One report states that only 2 percent of dogs have improved seizure control. Phenytoin has to be administered in high dosages every eight hours.

Dosage – It takes four to ten days to reach a state of concentration in the dog.

Side effect – Adverse effects in dogs include anorexia, vomiting, ataxia, and sedation. The combined use of phenobarbital with phenytoin increases the risk of liver disease.

Vigabatrin (Sabril)

Vigabatrin is a gamma-aminobutyric acid-transaminase (GABA-T) inhibitor that is effective in the treatment of certain types of drug-resistant or uncontrolled epilepsy but

is known to cause fluid on the brain (vacuolation) and lesions in the brains of treated dogs. It **has been evaluated in a small number of dogs with idiopathic epilepsy. Results were not very encouraging and several dogs developed hemolytic anemia that required stopping the drug.**

Oxcarbarepine (Trileptal)

Oxcarbarepine is an antiepileptic drug designed to reduce the impulses between the nerves that cause seizures. It does not affect the kidneys or the liver. The elimination half-life is approximately four hours. The very short half-life suggests oxcarbazepine is probably unsuitable as antiseizure medication in dogs.

Carbamazepine (Tegretol)

Carbamazepine is one of the most widely used antiseizure **drugs in people. Unfortunately, this drug is eliminated very quickly in dogs, with a half-life of only one to two hours compared to five to twenty-five hours in people. With long-term use, the half-life becomes even shorter because of increased liver metabolism.** Carbamazepine may be employed on its own or in combination with other anticonvulsants.

Dosage – The dosage in dogs varies and is adjusted to effect. Common dosages include the following: A. 2 to 6 mg/kg/day orally, divided and given over eight to twelve hours B. 4 to 8 mg/kg every twelve hours C. 15 to 20 mg per dog orally every twelve hours

Side effects – While generally safe and effective when prescribed by a veterinarian, carbamazepine may cause side effects in some dogs.

Zonisamide (Zonegran)

Zonisamide (zonegran) is an anticonvulsant medication which is used to stabilize electrical impulses in the brain, which can prevent seizures. Most vets prescribe phenobarbital or potassium bromide for a dog diagnosed with epilepsy or seizures, but if the dog does not react well with either of these drugs, the veterinarian may add zonisamide in combination with the drugs to treat the seizures.

How zonisamide works to prevent seizures is not known at this time, but it's believed that the medicine blocks sodium and calcium channels in the brain.

Zonisamide is metabolized by the liver, with a half-life of 15 hours and is eliminated through the urine. One of the problems with this drug is the cost and availability.

Dosage – The usual dosage for a dog with epilepsy is 11–22 mg/lb weight. It would be administered twice a day orally (every eight to twelve hours). Veterinarians usually chose the liquid formula of the drug but tablets are available.

Side effect – The most common side effects are drowsiness, loss of muscle control, vomiting, sedation, loss of appetite, loss of coordination, anorexia, and diarrhea. Zonisamide should not be given to pregnant dogs since it's known to cause birth defects in puppies.

Gabapentin (Neurontin)

Gabapentin is used to control or prevent seizures or convulsions and as a pain reliever.

This drug works by inhibiting calcium channels, thus preventing the calcium influx to cells that can cause seizures. The mechanism of action for pain control is not completely understood. Gabapentin is quickly absorbed and reaches peak affect in approximately two hours. Gabapentin has a short half-life of between two to four hours.

Dosage – For seizure treatment in dogs, gabapentin is stated at 5 to 10 mg per pound (10 to 20 mg/kf) every six to twelve hours. For dogs with cluster seizures, the dosage is 10mg/kg every eight hours for three days. Gabapentin should be given according to your veterinarian's instructions. The dose may be adjusted as necessary by your veterinarian depending on the response to the treatment.

Side effects – Side effects from gabapentin can include but are not limited to tremors, vomiting, drowsiness, loss of balance, and diarrhea.

Imepitoin (Pexion)

Imepitoin is an antiepileptic drug licensed in the European Union for the treatment of canine idiopathic epilepsy. **Imepitoin is one of a class of drugs called imidazolinone derivatives. These drugs are also known to be** anxiolytic**, That is, like valium** (*diazepam*)**, they are calming, so at higher doses or in highly susceptible individuals they might change a dog's behavior in variable ways.**

Dosage – Imepitoin (pexion) is given twice daily and acts rapidly to control seizures. It begins working in a few hours and after about three days a steady state has been achieved. The starting dose is normally 10–30 milligrams mg for every kilogram of body weight twice daily. A treatment with 30 mg/kg resulted in a significantly greater reduction in monthly seizure frequency relative to baseline data as compared to the 1 mg/kg dose. Both generalized and partial seizures but not cluster seizures were significantly less frequent in the high dose group. The dose required to control seizures varies greatly between individuals. Every dog breaks down and gets rid of the drug at a different rate. Imepitoin must be given every twelve hours, otherwise the concentration of drug in the blood may dip making your pet more prone to seizures. Imepitoin is best given on an empty stomach. What is most important is that it is given at a regular time each day so that doses are never forgotten.

Side effects – Some dogs will have a slight increased thirst or hunger, or be slightly sedated when they first start taking imepitoin. These effects are usually less obvious when compared with other treatments and tend to disappear anyway once a dog has adjusted to being on regular medication. Imepitoin does not cause the liver damage which has sometimes been associated with other treatments. Due to the mode of excretion, imepitoin is also safe for dogs with reduced kidney function.

Testing and Monitoring

Chemical Panel

It has been determined that 20 percent of the dogs on phenobarbital develop liver damage. It is very important to monitor your dogs' level of phenobarbital in your dogs' blood. This is done by having a laboratory test or chemistry panel of the liver enzymes, ALT, GGT, and alkaline phosphate every three to four months. This is vital to the health of any dog taking this antiseizure medication. Although with proper monitoring the risk of phenobarbital induced liver disease is low, the risk does exist. If all three liver enzymes are severely elevated (more than just a few points above normal), then you should do a urine bile acid test or a pre and post meal bile acid test to see what kind of damage has been actually done to the liver. You can change the diet to the liver cleansing diet and reduce the phenobarbital may regenerate the liver. Unfortunately when there are signs of liver disease, it may be too late.

Pre or Post Meal Bile Test

It is a hassle to do the pre- and post-bile acid testing. Your epileptic dog has to undergo fasting, and fasting is difficult for some seizure dogs. Go to the veterinarian for the first blood draw, feed 1/2 can of dog food, and wait two hours for the second blood draw, or leave your dog, and pick them up later. Bile acid testing should be done every six months to make sure that your dog is not developing liver dysfunction, which is a pre-curser to liver disease. Liver disease can only be detected by blood chemistries which include liver enzymes; liver dysfunction can only be detected by the bile acid test. Both tests are therefore necessary. But, you don't have to go through the pre and post bile acid testing, because a new testing procedure is now available that is less expensive and does not require fasting, nor a two-hour wait. The new test is called urine bile acids testing.

Urine Bile Acids Test

This new method of testing for liver dysfunction is as good if not better than the standard pre- and post-bile acid blood draws. This new test is less expensive, and the dog does not require fasting. All that is needed is a urine sample collected four to six hours after the dog has eaten. The veterinarian will give you a urine sample kit to collect a urine sample from your dog. You will need at least one table spoon of urine to take to your veterinarian. Getting the tablespoon of urine is no small task. You will have to use a small bowl or shallow pie tin and follow your dog around when outside to relieve him or herself. Once in the pan or bowl, transfer it to the sample kit and refrigerate until taking it or sending to the veterinarian or a testing lab facility.

Chapter 28

The Liver

Watch for the signs of liver disease or dysfunction with you epileptic or seizure dog. If your dog shows any signs of toxicity, like ataxia or wobbliness, you need to get the laboratory chemical panel. If the liver enzymes ALT, GGT, and alkaline phosphate are elevated and urine bile test is needed to assess the damage. Some of the symptoms of liver disease are chronic weight loss, pain in the abdomen, orange urine, yellowing of the eyes and/or skin (jaundice), loss of appetite, vomiting, diarrhea, constipation, gray feces, swollen belly, lethargy, pacing, increased water consumption urination, and seizures. If any of these symptoms occur, see your veterinarian.

Repairing the Liver

When liver damage has been determined by a urine bile acid test or a pre and post meal bile acid test, there is a number of things to do to reversing liver damage. Obviously, reduce the amount of drug dosage to be determined by your veterinarian. The best recommendation is to reduce the drugs 10 percent every three weeks.

This length is to avoid seizures from dropping the medication too quickly and too soon. Then start your dog on a liver cleansing diet to reverse the damage done.

Liver Cleansing Diet

When liver damage has been determined by the urine bile test, a liver cleansing diet should consist of home-cooked food and raw food. Fruits, low fat, white fish, and **vegetables** are an essential part of a liver cleansing diet. The diet should consist of 25% **fish** and 75% **vegetables** like **potatoes, sweet potatoes, zucchini, string beans,** and **squash**. Non**meat protein**s sources, such as **dairy products,** including cottage cheese, ricotta cheese, and yogurt, may be easier to digest and produce less ammonia than meat products. Look for low salt varieties if you feed a lot of cottage cheese, or if your dog will develop ascites (fluid retention). **Goat's milk** is easier for dogs to digest than cow's milk and **eggs, and they** are an excellent protein source for dogs with liver disease. The veterinarian can recommend an appropriate diet, which might include carefully regulated portions of certain **carbohydrates**, vitamins, proteins, minerals, and fats. The liver is unique since it has a large reserve capacity and more regenerative capability than almost any other organ. As a result, canine liver disease typically can be treated, or at least managed, if a diagnosis is made early enough. The goals of treating liver disease are to eliminate harmful toxins or minimize their detrimental effects on the liver, promote healing and regeneration of liver tissue, prevent or control complications of liver dysfunction, treat the underlying cause when possible, and keep the dog as comfortable and stable as possible until sufficient liver function can be restored. Treatment options include prescription and over-the-counter medications, dietary supplements, lifestyle changes, supportive care, surgical procedures, and a number of other possible therapies that the attending veterinarian will discuss with the dog's owner. The liver performs over 500 important functions. One of the most important is to filter and clean the blood of digestion byproducts like ammonia, toxins, and medications. The liver also regulates the iron level in the blood, which is critical to the blood's ability to carry oxygen throughout the body. Another critical function of the liver is to produce bile, which is necessary for the intestinal tract to process and digest food. When the liver is stressed, its cleaning and regulating capabilities often decrease or even stop. There is a possibility that certain fruits are liver protective, including watermelon, grapefruit, fig, kiwi, cherry, japanese plum, and papaya.

Remove Grains – One of the first steps in cleansing the liver is to remove grains from your dog's diet. Aflatoxin, a toxin from mold, is common in many grain crops, including corn, sorghum, millet, and soybeans. Even the small amounts of aflatoxin allowed in dog food can stress a dog's liver, and larger amounts can cause severe liver damage. Removing grains from your dog's diet allows the liver to try to cleanse itself of existing aflatoxin and stop any additional buildup of the toxin in the liver.

Replace Kibble – Dogs need protein to be healthy. The liver produces the bile needed to digest food in the intestinal tract. Dry kibble is the most difficult form of food for dogs to digest. Some studies have shown that kibble takes an average of twelve to fourteen hours to digest. Kibble with synthetic chemicals, additives, or byproducts can take as long as twenty-four to thirty-six hours. Replacing kibble in your dog's diet with canned food or raw food will significantly reduce digestion time, which means less bile is needed. The liver will not have to work as hard if your dog is on a more natural diet of canned or raw food, allowing it to better cleanse itself and perform its other necessary functions in the body.

Add Antioxidant Supplements – Adding a good supplement of antioxidants to your dog's diet can ease the stress on the liver and help remove toxins and free radicals from your dog's body. Vitamins A, B, C, E, K, zinc, adenosylmethionine (SAMe), trace minerals, and phosphatidylcholine (PC) will all help the body filter toxins, allowing the liver to cleanse itself more efficiently. Avoid supplements that contain copper or potassium, as these place more stress on the liver and any excess will build up. **Avoid supplements with copper and** foods that are high in copper, including most organ meats, especially beef liver (but not chicken or turkey liver, which have little copper); lamb, pork, duck, and salmon are high in copper; turkey, chicken, and other fish have moderate amounts of copper; and beef, cheese, and eggs are low in copper. In advanced stages of liver disease, both copper and sodium (salt) must be severely restricted; salt is restricted to help prevent ascites (fluid buildup in the abdomen) related to low albumin levels, which are caused by poor liver function. Of antioxidants, vitamin C could be the most important antioxidant for the liver. Even though dogs produce their own, a little extra help during a cleansing is prudent and easy. Whole food vitamin C from plant sources such as camu camu and acerola berries are very absorbable.

Zinc should be increased in above normal levels to help bind copper, and because its antioxidant properties help to protect the liver. **Vitamin A** should be limited with liver disease—normal amounts are fine, but don't give higher amounts. Cod liver oil, which is high in vitamin A, should be used sparingly, if at all, and liver should also be limited (liver is also high in copper). **Fish oil** can be given in moderate amounts, maybe 1000 mg per 20–30 lbs of body weight; it's not known whether it's helpful for liver disease or not but can help with inflammation. Current research indicates <u>SAMe</u> (S-Adenosyl-L-Methionine) may be beneficial for liver problems— give 200 mg twice a day to a large dog (recommended dosage is 10 mg per pound of body weight daily). SAMe is **best given on an empty stomach**, at least one hour before or two hours after eating (longer is better). If you have a small dog, you may need to use the veterinary drug **d**enosyl**,** which is also SAMe but comes in a 90 mg size (vetri-SAMe, sogeval and NOW brand offer 90–100 mg tablets). You can also give **d**enamarin, which is a combination of SAMe and milk thistle extract (silymarin).

Glutathione – Glutathione is a powerful antioxidant that is responsible for removing toxins, free radicals, and heavy metals that may pose risks and threats to the health of the body. It's estimated that up to 45% of liver disease in dogs is caused by low glutathione levels. S-adenosyl-L-methionine, also known as SAMe, is produced naturally in the body by amino acids and is another precursor to glutathione. SAMe improves detoxification, reduces inflammation, and serves as an antioxidant.

Milk Thistle

The most well-known herb of liver support is silymarin (milk thistle) for both humans and canines. Milk thistle is one of the very few traditionally used herbs that has been widely accepted by conventional science to have significant medicinal value. It has been called milk thistle because of a feature of the leaves, which are prominently splashed with white spots. This flower from the aster plant silymarin, protects the liver cells against toxins and their oxidative effects, helps regenerate liver cells, and stimulate protein synthesis. Milk thistle is a powerful antioxidant. Antioxidants protect us from chemicals in our bodies called free radicals. While we don't necessarily think of medications as toxins, many drugs and prescription medications can hurt the liver if taken in large enough doses or for long periods of time. Milk thistle can actually prevent or reduce medication induced liver damage. If you have been giving your pet medication and are concerned about the aftermath of chemicals residing in the body, milk thistle will help flush those out. If the liver has been weakened due to a bevy of reasons, it is unable to break down toxins. In order to combat allergens, the body produces histamine. The liver plays a role in this process: it removes the histamine from the body. If the liver is weakened and congested with toxins, the liver struggles and histamine builds up in the body, leading to more allergic reactions.

Dosage – The recommended dosage for **dogs** is 2 mg of **milk thistle** for each pound of dog weight.

Water

Give your dog clean filtered water to drink. Did you know that tap water contains a lot of toxins and by filtering the water we can eliminate up to 2100 known toxins?

The Detoxification Process

The chemicals and toxins built up in the liver are fat-soluble and is stored in the fat tissues of the liver. For the detoxification to work, there are two phases needed. In the first phase, there are certain nutrients that break down the toxins such as pollutants, insecticides, pesticides, drugs, food additive, and others. These nutrients are vitamins, antioxidants, folic acid, carotenoids, and natural herbs like milk thistle. The nutrients help to make the toxins become water soluble and ready to be eliminated from the liver.

The second phase is a group of nutrients such as amino acids, glutamine, glycine, taurine, cysteine, and sulphurated chemicals that work to eliminate the toxins from the liver by two ways. One way is through the kidneys as urine, the second is through the gall bladder as bile, and then eliminated through the bowels as excrement. If these nutrients are not balanced to support the detoxification, the breakdown of toxins in phase one will not be thorough (water-soluble) and/or the phase two of moving the toxins though the system to be eliminated will be blocked and clogged. After the detoxification has started, the dog may have some discharges that may occur naturally from the eyes, ears, and, nose. This is normal and results from inflammation due to the release of endotoxins as bacteria die off. Back off on the detox and things should correct.

Taurine and N-Acetylcysteine (NAC)

Traces of taurine may be present in pet foods, but it can be easily depleted in dogs who are stressed or with gastrointestinal issues. Taurine is also an antioxidant that has the ability to strengthen and stabilize cell membranes— making the cells more resilient to free radical attack. NAC is an antioxidant on a cellular level. It can bind heavy metals and has the ability to increase the levels of intracellular glutathione. Because of its expense to produce, n-acetylcysteine (NAC) and alpha lipoic acid serve as precursors for its production in the body. N-acetylcysteine can also fight infections and alpha lipoic acid can help regulate blood sugar and insulin levels.

Amino Acids

A high protein diet usually ensures the body of these protein building blocks; but a little more will ensure adequate detox flow. If your formula has taurine and glycine, it will be even better.

Liver Supplements

Note that many liver supplements contain similar ingredients, so if you give more than one at a time, you may be overdosing some things. For example, Liver Support Factors contains 100 mg of l-methionine per tablet, which is part of the s-adenosyl-methionine (SAMe) found in denosyl and SAMe supplements. Liver Support Factors also contains milk thistle (silybum marianum), which is included in <u>denamarin</u> (a combination of SAMe and the milk thistle extract silybin), and other liver support supplements. It would be better to rotate between different supplements rather than doubling up on some of these ingredients.

Flavonoids – Bioflavonoids such as from citrus, pycnogenol/pine bark, grape seed extract, green tea, quercitin, and rutin are important food-based nutrients that are best used as part of a detox combo formula.

Picrorhiza – an Ayurvedic (Indian) herb, has been shown to be even more effective than milk thistle for treating liver problems.

Korean red ginseng – has significantly improved liver function and accelerated regeneration of the liver in experimental dogs following partial hepatectomy (this is not the same as other forms of ginseng).

SBL Liv-T – is a homeopathic product from India. I was unable to get much information about this product from the company, and

I'm not a believer in homeopathy myself, but this may be worth trying based on the first-hand reports I've received of it helping dogs.

Prognosis

The liver is a remarkably complex organ that can malfunction and yet recover in multiple ways. Specific treatment protocols and an accurate prognosis depend almost entirely upon the cause and extent of liver dysfunction. Only a veterinarian can assess which treatment methods are best in any given case of canine liver disease, and provide an accurate prognosis for the dogs' path forward.

CHAPTER 29

Treatment with Diet

Healthy eating is key. You want to make sure your dog gets adequate nutrition. Depending on your dog's specific situation, sometimes diet changes alone can be effective in treating seizures. Numerous case studies have shown a correlation between food allergies and epilepsy. Switching your dog to a hypoallergenic diet or transitioning from an over-the-counter commercial food to home-prepared meals with organic ingredients can prevent seizures and make a huge difference in your dog's overall health.

Essential Fatty Acids (Omega 3 and Omega 6 oils) – Many humans with epilepsy have been helped by eating a Ketogenic diet (high in fat, low in carbohydrates). High fat seems to decrease the excitability of the neurons in the brain, and the addition of omega 3 and omega 6 fatty acids (both of which are found in wild-caught salmon oil) can decrease seizure frequency and intensity in dogs.

Consult with your veterinarian based on your dog's specific needs. Feed your dog a high-quality balanced diet with easily digestible protein (beef and fish are harder for dogs to digest), and no animal byproducts, fillers, or allergens.

Diet plays an important role in the management of canine epilepsy. It is very important to feed a kibble that is preservative-free. Preservatives such as ethoxyquin, BHT, and BHA should be avoided as they can cause seizures. Many supermarket dog foods are loaded with chemical dyes and preservatives. Buy a high-quality kibble made from good grain-free ingredients for your dog. If your dog is taking potassium bromide, be very careful when you switch dog foods. Try to make sure the sodium content is the same as the previous food. Change over very slowly, whether it is the same sodium content or different, so that the absorption rate of the potassium bromide remains the same. The best thing for your dog is fresh cooked or raw meals. Fresh meat or vegetables are good supplements to providing nutrients loss in the process of making kibbles in commercial dog foods. You may also choose a raw diet for your pet, including meats from trustworthy sources, vegetables, vitamins and mineral supplements. Raw meat is a quality, unaltered protein source. A lack of sufficient proteins and amino acids can cause a nutritional imbalance. Make sure that the diet you choose for your pet adheres to the principles of BARF.

When you change your dog's diet, you will have to take one to two weeks to make the transition. If the change is sudden, this may trigger seizures and digestive problems. Start by feeding the dog 25% of the ingredients from the new diet and 75% of the old one. Steadily increase the amount of ingredients from the new diet.

Do not consider changing your dog's diet without first understanding what a dog's diet should and should not include. For dogs on anti-epilepsy drugs, diet changes must be discussed with your veterinarian. Diet, drugs, canine metabolism, and the potential interactions must all be understood before changing anything in your dog's regimen.

The Raw Food Diet

Healthy Snacks

Include celery, carrots, apples, pears, bran crackers, rice cakes, peaches, hard-boiled eggs, scrambled eggs, oatmeal, cottage cheese, plain yogurt, homemade meatballs, chicken, bananas, dehydrated apricots, peanut butter, sweet potato, pumpkin, cucumbers, blueberries, and raspberries.

Nutraceuticals

A nutraceutical is a pharmaceutical grade and standardized nutrient. In the United States, nutraceuticals do not exist as a regulatory category; they are regulated as dietary supplements and food additives by the FDA under the authority of the Federal Food, Drug, and Cosmetic Act. A variety of vitamins and nutritional supplements have been highly effective in decreasing seizures in dogs. It is recommended to epileptic dogs: DMG (n dimethyl-glycine); choline; taurine; l-tryptophan; magnesium; melatonin; phosphatidylserine; and antioxidants such as vitamins C, A, and B complex.

Proteins

Dietary sources of high-quality animal proteins in the least processed forms provide the optimum amino acid profile for the canine. Commercial diets are generally measured by the quantity (percentage) of protein in the food. While protein content is important, the source of the protein is of greater importance. In a commercial dog food, protein is provided by combining animal sources (meat, byproducts, chicken, cheese, milk, fish, turkey or lamb) and grain sources (corn, wheat, rice and soy). The sum of these proteins appears on dog food packages as crude protein. Many amino acids are available only from animal protein sources, and if plant/vegetable/cereal/grain are the main protein sources, a dog may develop an animal protein deficiency. When the package lists these protein sources first in the ingredient list, or these sources dominate the first five items in the ingredient list, the food is most definitely deficient in animal protein. When heated, proteins are partially destroyed; all dry and canned commercial dog food is heated in the manufacturing process—so commercial food contains protein that is somewhat deficient or destroyed through heating. This protein deficiency in turn, results in deficiencies of amino acids, the building blocks the body requires to reconstruct proteins essential for health, including a healthy nervous system. In dogs with seizure disorders, there are deficiencies of proteins and amino acids.

Amino Acids

Diets deficient in amino acids, and chemicals that make up proteins, can significantly increase the possible risk of epileptic seizures in dogs. All amino acids are obtained from food. Taurine is an amino acids that is essential in the function of the nervous system. Dogs deficient in this amino acid are known to have seizures. Taurine is an amino acids that a dog can only produce if supplied adequate sources of animal protein containing the essential amino acids. There is evidence that it has a role in preventing seizures and liver disease, and also it can prevent diabetes and obesity in dogs as well as strengthening the heart and blood vessels. Taurine lowers the blood sugar levels, helps the body's consumption, and use of minerals such as sodium, calcium, zinc, and magnesium if deficiencies are implicated in seizures in dogs. Carnitine is a nonessential amino acid that takes fatty acids into the mitochondria (cells) where it can be burned up, used as fuel to reduce weight, and its deficiency is associated with epilepsy. Many other amino acid deficiencies are associated with seizure disorders. Amino acids operate in conjunction with each other, and with vitamins and minerals to ensure the body is supplied with the nutrients required for health.

Enzymes

An enzyme is a protein manufactured by a cell that speeds up the biochemical catalysts that converts one molecule into another. All living organisms have enzymes. They are involved in almost all bodily functions including the brain and nervous system. Any malfunction of a critical enzyme through mutation, underproduction, overproduction, or deletion can cause a genetic disease. The two main enzymes are metabolic and digestive.

Metabolic enzymes are produced internally by the body and are responsible for running the organs, blood, and tissue. Metabolic enzymes are needed to convert food into fuel for the cells in the body for growth, replacement, maintenance and repair.

Digestive enzymes are one of the most important facet in the body. The digestive enzyme is required for the breakdown of food, that contains the proteins, fats, and carbohydrates needed for fuel for the body. Digestion enzymes starts in the mouth, which triggers a release in the stomach and intestines. Nutrients from food require digestive enzymes to be absorbed into the bloodstream. Enzymes are found both in unprocessed foods, raw foods, and in the body itself. Dogs get enzymes from uncooked food like raw vegetables and fruit. The problem with most dog foods is that they are heated during the manufacturing process, thus killing enzymes, and force the body to provide all of the enzymes required to digest the food. When cooked/processed foods are consumed, the stomach recognizes that there are no enzymes in the cooked food and not enough enzymes in the stomach to break the food down; it will then signal the brain to send enzymes from other parts of the body, like the heart or liver. This is known as *enzyme robbing* and can be detrimental to the organs that are losing the enzyme causing the organs to be dysfunctional and diseased. Raw foods contain their own enzymes and eliminates the need for the stomach to request enzymes from other body organs to accomplish digestion. A canine diet rich in raw meat and plant material provides a good source of supplemental enzymes necessary for the continuing health of our dogs.

Vitamins

Vitamins are an organic compound and is essential for normal growth and development in a body. They are nutrients absorbed from food intake and react in the body to produce skin, organs, bone, and muscle. Most nutrients are found in natural foods and are in most commercially processed dog food. Because vitamins are destroyed by heat in the manufacturing process, dogs may need to have a vitamin supplement to maintain a healthy level of nutrients required to protect the dog from disease and dysfunction caused by a lack of vitamins. Also check the label on the food the dog is eating. Some commercial dog foods contain added vitamins as an ingredient to their foods, but those are not enough to make a difference due to state regulations. A prescribed dog food will have a therapeutic dose of vitamins and contain enough supplements to maintain a level of health. There are various vitamin deficiencies that are specifically linked to seizures in dogs.

Vitamin A

Vitamin A, also called carotene, is a fat-soluble antioxidant vitamin that is stored in the liver. It is needed for a dog's skin, coat, vision, muscles, and more, Sources of vitamin A include dairy products, fish oil, liver, dark fruits and vegetables, and egg yolks. The problem with vitamin A is that since it is fat-soluble and stored in the liver, excess vitamin A cannot be excreted or eliminated from the body like water-soluble vitamins, which means it can reach high toxic levels within the dog's body. Toxicity occurs usually when an owner feed their dog, usually puppies, supplemental vitamin A or too much fish liver oil. Symptoms of canine toxicity is weight loss, stiffness, lethargy, no appetite, and weakness.

Vitamin B

Vitamin B, is called B complex because it includes eight types. These are vitamin B1 (thiamine), vitamin B2 (riboflavin), vitamin B3 (niacin), vitamin B5 (pantothenic acid) vitamin B6 (pyridoxine), vitamin B7 (biotin), vitamin B9 (folic acid), and vitamin B12 (cobalamin). The vitamin B complex are water-soluble vitamins found in unprocessed foods and added to some commercial dog foods as a supplement. Check the label. Because the vitamin B complex is water-soluble, and excess vitamins are readily excreted out the body. An excellent source of **B** vitamins are turkey, tuna, liver, beans, and whole grains. Deficiency of vitamin B is well-known as a cause for seizures in canines, because commercial foods are cooked and would destroy these vital vitamins, either a raw diet or vitamin supplements are required especially for seizure dogs. Deficiency in vitamin B6 has been known to cause seizures in dogs, but an excess of vitamin B6 can cause ataxia (loss of balance) and possibly liver disease.

Vitamin C

Vitamin C also known as ascorbic acid is essential nutrient found in numerous fruits and vegetables such as apples, green beans, and sweet potatoes. Take note that you should not give a dog a whole apple since the seeds in the core contain cyanide and is poisonous. Dogs can produce vitamin C in their body from sun light, but if a dog is sick or stressed the dog can cause the depletion of vitamin C. Vitamin C is vital for dogs because it boosts the immune system, protects against numerous diseases, and gives the dog to recover from an injury or illness. It also acts as an anticarcinogen in dogs, protects against allergies, and helps in several bacterial or viral infections.

Vitamin D

Vitamin D is a fat-soluble vitamin like vitamin A that is stored in the liver and is vital for bone, nerve, and muscle health in your dog. It also regulates calcium in the kidneys and the body. High levels of vitamin D from drugs or diet can cause toxicity in dogs, and usually, the puppies are at a higher risk. One cause of vitamin D toxicity in dogs is the ingestion of rat poison chemicals.

Vitamin E

Vitamin E is an essential and important antioxidant that plays a crucial role in your dog's health. Vitamin E protects cells and helps cells repair damage caused by free radicals, a group of atoms produced by the body or an outside source, usually a toxin or pollutant. Most commercial dog food has the minimum amount of vitamin E needed to maintain healthy diet and a deficiency is rare in dogs. Vitamin E can be found in green leafy vegetables, and plant oils. Vitamin E deficiency is known to cause seizures and adding vitamin E as a supplement to a diet can reduce seizure frequency in dogs afflicted with epilepsy.

Minerals

The presents of minerals in dogs are essential for health, and play an important part in a dog's nutrition. Minerals aid in the formation of bone, oxygen in the blood, and normal muscle and nerve function. Minerals are divided in to two groups: the high-quantity group, known as macrominerals are calcium, phosphorus, potassium, sodium, and magnesium. The low-quantity group, which is known as microminerals (trace minerals) are: selenium, manganese, zinc, copper, iron, chromium and iodine. The macrominerals are required in greater amounts in a dog's body, while the microminerals are needed in smaller quantities. Deficiency in minerals in dogs can cause anemia, dehydration, and may lead to more serious health conditions. Mineral deficiency are known to cause or aggravate seizures in dogs. Most commercial dog food contains the minimum daily amount for dogs, but every dog is different in age, breed, size, metabolism, and activity level, which will require a higher need for additional minerals. For these dogs, a nutritional supplement should be considered. Always ask your veterinarian to assess your dog's needs, and recommend a good supplement.

Iron

The most common deficiency in dogs is iron, and iron is needed in the formation of red blood cells. Without iron, a canine will develop anemia. The cause for iron deficiency can be blood loss, tumors, parasites, lymphoma, or urinary tract infection. Symptoms could be lethargy, rapid breathing, depression, anorexia, disease prone, depression, and weakness.

Magnesium

Magnesium is a key nutrient mineral involved in energy production at a cellular level to move muscles and transfer the energy where it's required as well as for proper bone growth. It is needed for the absorption of certain other minerals and vitamins. It is the second most abundant mineral in a dog's body. Magnesium can be found in milk, fish, whole grains, soybeans, and wheat germ, although cooking can remove the mineral from the food. Magnesium is the second most abundant substance in cells next to potassium, so a deficiency in magnesium is a serious health concern. In the body, 60 percent of magnesium is found in the bones, and 40 percent is found in the liver and soft tissue. Magnesium deficiencies are rare, and are mostly due to malnutrition. It's symptoms are muscle tremors, weakness, depression, incoordination, lethargy, and then seizures.

Manganese

Manganese occurs mostly in a dog's liver but can be found in the kidneys, pancreas, and bone. It is needed for the proper use of protein and carbohydrate by the body and the maintenance of the nervous system. Manganese deficiency is rare in dogs, but if it occurs, it's usually with newborn or puppies and its symptoms include ataxia (loss of equilibrium), poor growth, and eventually, seizures. Good sources of manganese are whole grains, eggs, nuts, and green vegetables.

Selenium

Selenium is an antioxidant, which in conjunction with vitamin E and enzymes, protect the cells in the body from cancer, aging, fighting inflammation, and maintaining thyroid hormone levels. Food sources of selenium are wheat germ, bran, brown rice, oats, tuna fish, liver, turnips, and barley. An important factor of concern is that in some farms, the soil many be deficient in selenium and vegetables grown in that soil will not have the mineral selenium in the vegetable. Selenium deficiency in dogs are rare but is often prescribed as an antioxidant for dogs with epilepsy, inflammatory bowel disease, and cancer.

Calcium

Calcium is beneficial in dogs for bone growth, nails, teeth, and their coat. Without calcium, a dog is more susceptible to osteoporosis, bone diseases, and heart problems.

Calcium can be found in milk, yogurt, cottage cheese, and cheese. Other source are fish, salmon, tuna, sardines, and trout cooked (never raw). Do not feed your dog bones even though they are rich in calcium, a splinter can puncture an organ resulting in death. Symptoms for a calcium deficiency is rickets, muscle twitching, lethargy, panting, stiffness, and seizures.

Zinc

Zinc is an essential mineral that is critical for canine body function, particularly the skin and coat. Beside supporting the immune system and improving energy this nutrient is good for a dogs general health. Zinc is found in oysters, and to a far lesser degree in most animal proteins, beans, nuts, almonds, whole grains, pumpkin seeds and sunflower seeds, but studies show up to 40% of zinc intake is not used by the body.

There is a fragile balance on how much zinc a dog needs to have. An excess of Zinc and the dog will develop zinc toxicity. Symptoms include jaundice, depression, lethargy, diarrhea, vomiting, and lack of appetite. Causes of this usually is swallowing a toy from a board game, pennies, nails, staples, and some lotions. Too little zinc and the regeneration of hair, skin, nails, and general healing if reduced. The best advice is to ask a veterinarian to test your dog's blood, and see what the diagnoses is, and recommend a course of action—either a zinc supplement or a blood transfusion.

Ingredients to Avoid

Find a dog food that is not manufactured using artificial preservatives such as **BHA** (butylated hydroxyanisole or E 320) and **BHT** (butylated hydroxytoluene or E321), or other colorants and artificial flavors. Gluten (which may be found in grains), rye, barley and oats, which are known to arouse the opiate receptors in the brain; thus, seizures are more likely to occur. Complex carbohydrates could cause hyperglycemia. Hyperglycemia may trigger a seizure. Soy products, casein, corn, and dairy products are examples. Foods and treats with a lot of salt can actually cause your dog to have a seizure if they are on potassium bromide, so cut them out of the diet.

CHAPTER 30

Natural, Homeopathic, and Holistic Treatment

I. Natural Treatments

The use of natural remedies has existed long before written history. Before modern medicine, natural treatments were the only way to help with ailments and diseases. The emergence of pharmaceutical companies has deterred the use of natural remedies, but they remain beneficial and should remain an important aspect in today's modern age. Natural treatments are cost-effective and easy to administer in your home. Natural remedies are safe and less likely to cause complications. Many of these natural treatments have been used for hundreds, if not thousands of years, and because of this their safety and potential side effects are well known. This is compared to the short term testing, often only weeks, that is carried out by pharmaceutical companies, and many prescription drugs hit the market with their long-term consequences unknown. Some of the most dangerous chemicals and substances that Americans consume are through the use of prescriptions. Seizures leave your pet tired and weak because of the movement and jerks they make during the episodes. Dog seizures can happen more than once in a day depending on the extent of damage caused in the pet's body. Pets can get dog seizures due to injuries and growth in their brains.

Here are some of the ways you can use to treat seizures in dogs naturally.

Vitamins (Nutraceuticals)

Some dogs are affected by seizures when their bodies lack vitamins. You should get vitamin **supplements** to suppress the fits. Even humans suffer from seizures when their bodies lack vitamins. The use of vitamins will help improve the health of your pet. This is also covered under the information in holistic.

Diet Change

You need to check the food that you give your pet every day. Some of the foods can cause an allergic reaction to your pet. An elimination diet can help you identify the foods which cause seizures in your **pet**. There are commercial foods which are hypo allergenic and contain no preservatives. They can help you treat seizures in your pet. Also, make sure that if you decide to make food for your pet at home, it should be a balanced diet. This too is covered in chapter 29.

Environmental Pollutants

If your pet suffers from seizures and epileptic attacks, you should keep it in a clean environment. Do not use anything which pollutes the air. Most of the chemicals used in various ways at home can trigger **seizures in dogs.** Do not use strong pesticides for your garden and flowers. Some of the air fresheners and cleaning detergents are also bad if your pet is allergic to chemicals. Try to use friendly pesticides and soaps in your home. Give your pet pure drinking water which does not contain fluoride or chlorine.

Fatty Acids

You should give your dog salmon oil every day. This ensures that your pet remains healthy. Other oils like flax seed and primrose also give your pet fatty acids which are essential for your pet's health.

Cooling down the Dog

During a seizure, the dog can overheat due to hyperthermia (high body temperature), and this can cause brain damage, so it's important to keep your pet cool during a seizure. One of the ways to reduce the core temperature is to apply a cool wet towel to the dog's paws and chest, refreshing the towel every few minutes. Another is to use a washcloth or sponge to wet the fur. Placing a fan near the dog at low speed will also cool the dog. Do not submerge a dog in water because this can cause the dog to go into shock.

Applying Ice

A new technique being used to reduce the duration of a seizure is to apply ice pack or a bag of ice to the lower midsection of your dog's back and holding the bag firmly in position until the seizure ends. The exact area on the back is between the 10th thoracic (chest) and 4th lumbar (lower back) vertebrae (bones in the spine); what this means is that the top of the ice bag should rest just above the middle of your dog's back, following along the spine, and drape down to the lower midsection of the back. You don't have to be exact, just figure on the middle of the back, and the area will be covered. You should have the ice ready and prepared in the freezer. If you have a small dog, fill a small-sized (quart) Ziploc freezer bag with cubed or crushed ice and keep it in a particular spot in your freezer. If you have a large dog, use a large-sized (gallon) bag. Remove the ice when the seizure is over. The use of ice can help to shorten the epileptic episodes.

Sugary foods

A seizure makes your pet get low sugar levels in its blood. You need to boost it by giving it things like honey or any other sweet foods. If you leave it without replacing sugar in its body, it will suffer another fit.

II. Holistic Treatments

Holistic is a form of healing that considers the whole person (or dog, in this case) body, mind, spirit, and emotions in the quest for optimal health and wellness. According to the holistic medicine philosophy, one can achieve optimal health, the primary goal of holistic medicine practice, by gaining proper balance in life.

Holistic medicine practitioners believe that the whole person is made up of interdependent parts, and if one part is not working properly, all the other parts will be affected. In this way, if dogs have imbalances (physical, emotional, or spiritual) in their lives, it can negatively affect their overall health. A holistic doctor may use alternative treatments, and they include homeopathic remedies, herbal medicine, as well as acupuncture. Holistic medicine for dogs and homeopathy are always used as an alternative therapy to conventional medications.

Holistic veterinarians look for ways to treat seizures as an alternatives to anticonvulsant medication, which can have toxic side effects and cause over sedation and personality changes when used on prolonged basis. Natural therapies don't usually lead to side effects or require the same intense regimen of regular evaluation.

Acupuncture

Acupuncture is a practice of inserting small needles into the skin at specific points called acupoints to alleviate pain, treat disease, improve function, or a treat a medical condition. Acupuncture originated in China over 5000 years ago, and is popular in the west with trained and licensed medical doctors using acupuncture with western medicine to give the patient the most benefit for the treatment of an illness. Acupuncture is a technique for balancing the flow of the life force known as chi or qi (chee) that flows through pathways called meridians. Acupuncturist believe the energy flow can be rebalanced by inserting needles along a meridian. There is very low risk using acupuncture on your dog if you have a certified competent acupuncturist. Veterinary acupuncturists use transpositional points, the locations of which are transposed to canines from the human acupoints. The treatment of dogs with acupuncture is mainly for neurological conditions such as seizures or epilepsy, but can be used for other medical or health conditions.

Acupressure

Acupressure is an ancient traditional Chinese medicine art that can be thought of as *acupuncture without needles.* Like human acupressure, animal acupressure stimulates or sedates points lying along the energy channels known as meridians, moving the energy, balancing the chi, and relieving or preventing blockages and excesses that can cause discomfort, pain, and disease.

Aromatherapy

Aromatherapy is gaining popularity as a safe and effective alternative treatment to tackle dog health problems. Aromatherapy uses aromatic plant oils or essential oils as a treatment to prevent disease, reduce pain, induce relaxation, and anxiety. There is evidence that aromatherapy can reduce stress and improve the general well-being of a dog, but no medical evidence that it can cure any disease.

Aquapuncture

Aquapuncture is the injecting of a solution of vitamin B12 and saline into the acuapuncture points of a dog along a meridian. The solution will be absorbed slowly and thus stimulates the point for a longer period of time.

Electroacupuncture

Developed in China in 1934, as an improvement over conventional acupuncture. Electroacupuncture is a form of acupuncture where a small electric current is passed through two acupuncture needles at an acupoint on a meridian. This treatment is especially good at reducing pain and can restore a dogs well-being by encouraging the flow of energy.

Laser Acupuncture

This uses lasers rather than needles on acupoints and is very cool and does not generate much heat. This is great for dogs who absolutely don't tolerate needle insertions.

Chiropractic Care

Regular chiropractic adjustments are especially effective in treating cases of epilepsy that follow head injuries or physical trauma, as well as chronic, recurrent ear infections that seem to trigger seizures. Make sure your pet's chiropractor is a certified veterinary chiropractor with experience in canine epilepsy.

Nutraceuticals

A variety of vitamins and nutritional supplements have been highly effective in decreasing seizures in dogs. It is recommend the following for epileptic dogs, DMG (n dimethyl-glycine); choline; taurine; l-tryptophan; magnesium; melatonin; phosphatidylserine; and antioxidants such as vitamins C, A and B complex.

Western Herbs

Herbs contain numerous chemical constituents, which can have medicinal effects on our pets' bodies. When used appropriately, the medicinal properties of specific herbs can regulate and normalize specific activities of one or more organ systems. Herbs have been used by people since thousands of years ago. Many animals, including our pets, instinctively feed on certain types of plants when they are suffering from, say, indigestion or upset stomach. Herbs usually act much more slowly than Western medicines so do not expect any quick-fix from herbal treatments. In general, it takes at least sixty to ninety days after the beginning of herbal treatments to see any significant improvement in a pet's health conditions.

While herbs are, in many ways, better and gentler to our pets than conventional medicines, it is not advisable to use herbs in the place of veterinarian consultation, particularly in the event of a serious or life-threatening condition. In general, herbs are best used to support and improve the general physical well-being of our pets. Also, herbs are best used for treating chronic diseases and are not the preferred means of treatment in emergency situations. It is important that we obtain the best quality herbs from reputable and trustworthy suppliers. There are many over-the-counter western herbs, in both capsule and tincture form including:

Passion Flower – is good when you want calm a stressed pet down. By reducing anxiety and stress and reduce chances of any **seizures.**

Basil – This leafy herb has antioxidant, antiviral, and antimicrobial properties.

Parsley – A leafy herb commonly seen as a garnish on our plates is a source of flavonoids, antioxidants, and vitamins. It also contains lycopene and carotenes. Used to soothe the stomach, parsley has a long history of use with dogs.

Kiva – is used as a mild tranquilizer for anxiety in dogs.

Chamomile – a natural sedative that reduces anxiety and induces sleep.

Milk Thistle – (silymarin) this herb has significant medicinal value for protecting the liver and the supporting the immune system.

Skullcap – The herb commonly serves to calm nervous or irritated dogs and to help those recovering from surgery or trauma and is used to treat epilepsy.

Valerian – used as a sedative for spasms, convulsions and hyperactivity.

Oat straw – contains proteins, saponins, flovonoids, vitamins B1, B2, D, E, and carotene, and carries antispasmodic properties.

Rosemary –This herb is high in iron, calcium, and vitamin B6. Rosemary has also been shown to act as an antioxidant.

Oregano – oregano is high in antioxidants and flavonoids and is reported as an antimicrobial. This nontoxic herb has been used to help with digestive problems, diarrhea, and gas. Research using oil of oregano has also shown antifungal properties.

These herbs are all used to treat seizures. As with nutraceuticals, always discuss appropriate herbs and dosages with your veterinarian before giving them to your dog.

Chinese Herbs

In Traditional Chinese Veterinary Medicine, seizures and epilepsy belong to *Nei-feng* (Internal Wind) syndrome. The earliest literature on Internal Wind can be found in *Su Wen* published during the third century BC.

Ginkgo is an herbal remedy made from the leaf of the ginkgo tree, *ginkgo biloba*, is one of the oldest species of tree in the world. While the ginkgo nut is used in Chinese medicine in the treatment of respiratory disorders, the ginkgo leaf is used in Western herbal medicine, primarily to stimulate blood flow, both peripheral to the extremities and cerebral (to the brain). In dogs, ginkgo is most commonly recommended for the treatment of cognitive disorder brought on by senility.

Bupleurum – is effective in calming down the nervous system. Ancient Chinese medical texts dating back to two millennia mention the use of the bupleurum as an herbal tonic for the treatment and strengthening of the liver.

Di Tan Tang – is a Chinese herb that treats seizures and epilepsy in dogs.

Long Dan Xie Gan Tang – is a Chinese herb famous for its popular use in purging and cleansing the liver.

Ban Xie Zhu Tian Ma Tang – is a Chinese medicine that is used for the syndrome that includes vertigo, nausea, frequent headaches, and epilepsy.

Tian Ma Gou Teng Yin – this cleans the and quickens the blood, and supplements; it also boosts the liver and kidneys

San Ren Tang – it drains dampness from the lungs.

Bu Yang Huan Wu Tang – is an ancient Chinese herbal medicine that tones *Qi*, invigorates blood, and relieves the symptoms of ataxia and neuropsychiatric disorders, including a variety of neuralgias, epilepsy, and neuroses.

Magnets

Magnetic Therapy (or Magnetic Field Therapy) is used extensively in dogs to treat for medical conditions. Magnets, through a magnetic field helps the body at a cellular level by influencing the ion exchange at the cell. This can improve oxygen and induce repairs of damaged or diseased cell tissue. The use of magnets as a medical treatment can be traced to China in 2000 B.C. as well as ancient Egypt and Greece. Magnetic field therapy helps the body to heal by creating a favorable environment for repair. Magnets increase blood flow to the area, and bring in essential nutrients, and help relieve pain and inflammation. There are two types of magnet field therapy. The first uses permanent magnets to generate a magnetic field, and the second type uses pulse electromagnetic field (**PEMF**) a machine that generates a pulse of electromagnetic energy to the area of the injury or affliction. As with so many areas of alternative medicine, dog owners should always consult with an experienced veterinarian who is experienced with magnetic field therapy before deciding on this therapy and should always be administered by a trained therapist or veterinarian.

Essential oils

Essential oils have been around and used for thousands of years for medical purposes. An essential oil is a concentrated liquid substance that contains a part of a plant like the leaves, stems, flowers, fruit, seeds, resins, roots, peels, or bark. The plant will have a particular and unique aroma or fragrance that will become the essence of that plant. To get the oil of the plant or essence, an extraction process must be done, usually by distillation, but also can be done by solvent-extraction or cold pressing. Essential oils are highly concentrated and can cause an allergic reaction or skin irritation if used without dilution. The essence should be diluted with a common oil such as vegetable, olive, jojoba, or coconut.

Each essential oil has its own scent, color, chemical properties, and can have a health benefit. Many of the oils are antiviral, antifungal, antibacterial, detoxifying and anti-inflammatory.

On a physical level, many essential oils are antibacterial, antiviral, antifungal, anti-inflammatory, and detoxifying properties that help fight infections and strengthen your immune system. Other essential oils like peppermint can be a sedative and produce a calm relaxing feelings, while essential oils for stimulating are citrus, rosemary, jasmine, mint, eucalyptus, and others.

Essential oils are highly concentrated and therefore extremely potent. When using essential oils on our dogs; therefore, we should be careful not to overuse them. Always dilute essential oils with a carrier oil (such as olive oil, sweet almond oil, etc.) before use. If we choose essential oils that are safe for dogs, and use them in diluted form, they are can have a positive therapeutic effect. The oils commonly are applied to the skin where they are absorbed. They can be applied by massaging or petting your dog, or sprayed on with a spritzer bottle. Other methods is to use an inhaler or diffuser where the dog inhales the essential oils.

Frankincense – is the essential oil of choice for any kind of brain disorder. Frankincense has a molecular makeup that includes sesquiterpenes that is able to cross the blood/brain barrier. These sesquiterpenes stimulate the limbic system of the brain and other glands within the brain, promoting memory and releasing emotions. Frankincense slows down and deepens the breath. The therapeutic properties of Frankincense oil are antiseptic, astringent, carminative, cicatrisant, cytophylactic, digestive, diuretic, emmenagogue, expectorant, sedative, tonic, uterine, vulnerary, and expectorant.

Cardamom – is a diuretic, antibacterial, and normalizes appetite. It can cause colic, coughs, heartburn, and nausea.

Chamomile – There are two types of chamomile essential oil: German and Roman. German chamomile has anti-inflammatory benefits which can be good

for your dog's skin and coat; it may help to reduce allergic reactions. Roman chamomile helps to calm nerves and it may also reduce teething pain, cramps, and muscle pain.

Fennel – assists the adrenal cortex, helps break up toxins and fluid in tissue, balances pituitary, thyroid, and pineal glands.

Geranium – repels ticks and destroys bacteria.

Ginger – pain relief, nontoxic, good for motion sickness and digestion.

Helichrysum – antibacterial, reduces bleeding in accidents, skin regenerator, helps repair nerves; also useful in cardiac disease.

Lavender – essential oil, can be used pure or diluted; it is useful in conditioning patients to a safe space. May help allergies, burns, ulcers, insomnia, car ride anxiety and car sickness, to name a few.

Marjoram – Marjoram is a perennial herbal plant that has been as a culinary herb, medicine and fabric dye since ancient times. The Greeks used marjoram as an ingested and topical medicine. Marjoram contains multiple volatile oils that give the plant its medicinal properties that are antibacterial, anticarcinogen, antifungal, anti-inflammatory, antioxidant, antiseptic, and antispasmodic.

Niaouli – antihistaminic, powerful antibacterial properties.

Pepperment – This essential oil is an antispasmodic; it also helps to stimulate circulation which can benefit your dog's skin and coat. Peppermint essential oil can treat motion sickness, arthritis, and it can even repel insects.

Sweet Orange – Calming, deodorizing, flea repelling.

Spearmint – Helps to reduce weight, good for colic, diarrhea, nausea, helps balance metabolism, and stimulates gallbladder.

Vetiver – is known to have a calming cooling affect as it clears heat from the body and removes anxiety and restlessness.

Note: Some essential oils, diluted or not, are unsafe for dogs and use of such oils should be avoided altogether. Here are some essential oils that should not be used on dogs; anise, birch, bitter almond, calmus, camphor, cassia, chenopodium, clover leaf and bud, garlic, goosefoot, horseradish, hyssop, juniper, mugwort, mustard, pennyroyal, horseradish, rue, santalina, sassafras, savory, thyme, thuja, tansy, terebinth, wintergreen, wormwood, and yarrow.

Flower Essences – the Bach flower essence Rescue Remedy can be used when you suspect your dog is about to have a seizure or as an overall stress reducer to prevent future seizures.

Gold Beading

Gold bead implants are a permanent form of acupuncture. The gold beads are implanted on the acupuncture points on the dog's back and head. The gold beads are very tiny and about the size of a pinhead or tip of a fine ball point pen. They provide a long-term stimulation of the points. This form of treatment was pioneered in the 1970s. As with all forms of treatment, it will work for some and not for others. The first gold bead implants performed in the US were done in the early 1970s by Dr. Grady Young. Dr. Terry Durkes in Marion, Indiana began doing clinical research on using the implants in 1975, and initially used them to treat seizure disorders. Using a needle, three gold beads are implanted in each location, and the location is very precise. If the beads are off even one sixteenth of an inch (slightly less than 1.6 mm), they will not be successful.

People have reported that their dogs have bled at the locations where the gold beads were implanted, and this is a good sign. From the Chinese medicine perspective, seizures can be caused by too much internal heat, often from the liver, which creates wind and seizures are a symptom of the excess wind. When bleeding occurs where the beads are implanted, this means that the excess heat is being released. This makes it likely that the implants was needed in that area.

Gold is used because it is nonreactive with the body. It is not known exactly how the gold bead implants work, but it is thought that the gold beads emit a minute electrical charge, and the points that respond well to the implants have excessive negative charges.

III. Homeopathic Treatments

Homeopathic remedies work on the premise of *like cures like*. They contain tiny amounts of substances that, if given to a healthy animal, would cause symptoms similar to those you are treating. Perhaps one of the greatest assets of homeopathy is its ability to treat seizures. Choosing the perfect remedy for your pet's illness is a complicated process and requires an experienced homeopath; however, once a proper remedy is given, it can stop a seizure in its tracks. Commonly prescribed remedies include Belladonna, Aconitum and, in cases of vaccine-related seizures, Thuja. Seizures and epilepsy are typically the result of chronic, long standing disease and this makes the choice of remedy difficult. Consult with your homeopathic veterinarian to find the proper constitutional

Aconite – Aconite is for fear, anxiety and restlessness induced by shock, either physical or emotional trauma.

Belladonna – Belladonna is one of the few medicines for focal seizure. Belladonna works on your dog to **control seizure**, reduce its impact and time, **soothes your dog**, and controls the situation pretty well. Once medicated, the dog tends to go into a calm state and sometimes curls up to a nap.

Cocculus – is an excellent medication for dogs that travel a lot and are inclined to develop motion sickness. In addition, this remedy also aids in treating fatigue. A very useful remedy, its connection with vertigo gives it its place in this context.

Kali brom – Used as a conventional anticonvulsant.

Silica – having both convulsions and ailments from vaccination in its picture, is extremely useful when seizures are vaccine induced.

Lavender – reduces anxiety in dogs and boosts the immune system. **Taurine** – an amino acid used as an anticonvulsant for seizures in dogs.

Important!

Don't try giving these remedies to your dog unless you discuss these remedy choices with your homeopathic veterinarian before treating your dog. Seizures and epilepsy are typically the result of chronic, long standing disease, and this makes the choice of remedy difficult. Consult with your homeopathic veterinarian to find the proper constitutional. Unlike conventional medicines, homeopathy won't contribute to your dog's toxin buildup, and this gives him the very best chance of saying goodbye to seizures forever.

CHAPTER 31

Treatment of Status Epilepsy

Status epilepsy is a special case where seizure occurs longer than twenty minutes or two or more seizures lasting at least five minutes occurring without full recovery of consciousness or without abatement. If these seizures are not stopped, the resultant hypoxia may result in irreparable brain damage. Although status epilepsy is primarily a central nervous system abnormality, it results in significant systemic physiological changes. This differs from cluster seizures, in that the two or more seizures occur within a twenty-four-hour window, and the dog regains consciousness between seizures.

Immediate aggressive treatment is necessary to stem any neurological damage or death.

First, Call your Veterinarian immediately. A dog in status needs to get to a pet hospital or a vets care as soon as possible to prevent any damage. Status epilepticus, if untreated, may lead to death from hyperthermia (high body temperature), hypoxia (reduced blood flow to the organs) or circulatory and respiratory collapse. Have a plan for an in home emergency for this.

Second, Administer Valium. Try to stop the seizures. If this is not the first seizure your dog had, then you should be prepared ahead of time with an emergency medical kit. Your veterinarian can help assembly what you need for this kit. This requires diazepam (valium) injectable solution to be administered rectally, and is usually with a urinary catheter. Valium given rectally starts to be effective within minute and will last thirty to sixty minutes, compared to oral tablets that take thirty to sixty minutes to become effective, lasting one to two hours. The dosage to be administered is different for each dog depending on their size, medication history, and medical history. Your veterinarian will instruct you on the proper dosage to administer to your dog. Some dogs have an abnormal reaction to valium that makes them extremely agitated. If this is your case, your veterinarian can recommend other medications or combinations of medications that may be used to treat status epilepsy. Please ask your veterinarian for rectal and oral valium kit to have at home just in case your dog clusters or goes into status. Status is life-threatening and liquid injectable valium should stop status. It may save you a trip to the emergency room, and can possibly save your dog's life by the wait while driving to the veterinarian or animal hospital to stop the seizures. Follow the storage instructions for the valium in the kit from your pharmacist. This is usually a cool dry place.

Third, cool the body. Dogs can overheat during a seizure. Use a cool wet towel on your dog's chest and paws helps reduce his core temperature. Be sure to refresh the towels every few minutes. Also placing a fan on low speed will help cool your dog.

Forth, Get to the veterinarian or pet hospital for further treatment. Short-acting anaesthetic drugs like propofol are the most commonly used agents for treating resistant status epilepsy as they have a rapid onset of action, short half-lives, and reduce cerebral metabolic rates. These drugs should be used only in an intensive care setting because of the need for continuous blood pressure monitoring and ideally, central venous pressure monitoring. General anesthesia prevents tonic-clonic movements and allows manual control of respiration. Please remember that in the emergency room, if seizures continue, you could suggest using an IV valium drip (valium given intravenously), or even the mild anesthetic propofol, which is recommended for *epi's* to keep them sedated to break the cluster cycle. This anesthetic is the safest for seizures. Pentobarbital is not recommended as an anesthetic for dogs with epilepsy. After a severe seizure, you should always check your dog's gums. If they are pale or white, you need to get to an emergency room immediately. This could be pulmonary edema. Status epilepsy is a life-threatening situation, and the pet should be admitted to a medical facility for drug and fluid administration and profession treatment as soon as possible. Your main concern is to stabilize your dog for the trip to the medical facility.

The pet may need seven to ten days before returning to normal after a status epileptic prolonged seizure.

PART IV

THE CAREGIVER & PROGNOSIS

Chapter 32

The Caregiver

There is not a more selfless task as to caring for a dog you love—a dog in seizure. The responsibilities are overwhelming and very stressful. Just knowing that your helpless pet is relying on you and you alone for the normal thinks a dog needs like food, play, love, and companionship. Now, you need to maintain medication, special diet, constant monitoring, and the stress that goes with the worries of costs, daily doses of pills, veterinarian visits, and knowing that any minute of the day or night, the dreaded seizure may occur and you're up to the task of helping your best friend. You know your dog gives you unconditional love. Even as he or she has this horrible affliction, your dog will come out of the fog of a seizure and seek you out to lick your hand and face. Being your companion is their sole purpose in life. Those who never owned a dog will never understand. Your dog is your friend, your companion, playmate, guard dog, and alarm clock. Your dog is always fateful and never holds a grudge. But you, the caregiver, are his guardian angel.

What to do as a caregiver

1. **Investigate.** It is important that you learn as much as you can about canine epilepsy treatments and what is available to you. **Read up on canine seizures and canine epilepsy**

as much as you can, so you can make intelligent decisions on what to do, and prepare for seizures. Be open to alternative medicine and methods. Keep an open mind as to a possible treatment for your dog and remember anything you can do to slow, or stop a seizure and benefit your dog is good. New ideas and methods are being discovered and today may be the day a cure is found. Look on the Internet for site regarding **canine seizures or canine epilepsy.** There is a lot of information out there. Join a blog and exchange information with other canine pet owners who have seizure dogs. Get on a canine epilepsy or seizure mailing list. Listen and learn. Write down anything you feel is important to help your pet.

Keep a Log – Take notes of every seizure. Write down what your pet was doing before a seizure and how was the dog acting. What was the dog's environment like— loud music or on the lawn with weed killer? Writing this information down may help find specific triggers to a seizure. Note what the dog did during the seizure to determine the type of seizure for the veterinarian's information, especially if it was his first one. Also write down what transpired after the seizure. The log book should have the following information:

1. Date, and time.
2. Severity and length of time of the seizure.
3. Medications given, if any, to cope with the seizure, **or the** alternative such as ice packs or wet towels.
4. What your dog was doing prior to the seizure.
5. Any detail of the dog's behavior during the recovery from the seizure.

In your log note veterinarian visits, vaccination shots given, weather at the time, food changes, household cleaning done with chemicals, or medication given to the dog, daily amounts, and dosage. Keep a record of all the veterinarian lab tests done and the results, so the information can be shared with an alternative holistic veterinarian or neurologist if you desire. This historical information of your pet's seizures should be shared with your veterinarian during office visits so you don't have to rely on your memory of a seizure event and what transpired. Another record is to film the seizure on your cell phone to show your veterinarian.

2. **Testing** – After the first seizure, you need to have the dog tested for possible causes. This is a way to eliminate a variety of afflictions that can be detected by blood tests, urine tests, MRIs or X-rays. It may be that you will never know what the cause is, but to know what it is not, narrows the field of potential causes.
3. **Medication** – Look at the standard medications most veterinarians prescribe: phenobarbital and potassium Bromide. Are you willing to accept the side effects from this medication?
Will an alternative medication such as keppra, primidone, gabapentin, zonisamide, or a new European drug Pexion suffice? What about alternative medicines such as natural, holistic, or homeopathic?
4. **Lifestyle changes** – Look around the dogs environment and see what can be causing seizures. Examine his world and see what may be setting off a seizure. It could be anyone of causes list in Part II of this book.
5. **Diet**– Is the dog's food safe? Check the ingredients for chemicals and preservatives that can cause seizures. Look at natural foods as noted in chapter 15 and other foods not to feed your pet as noted in chapter 20.
6. **Be Prepared** – Keep phone numbers to your veterinarian and all emergency veterinarian hospitals near all phones or in your cell phone. Know the locations of the hospitals and the route to the facility. Have an emergency Valium kit available

in case of a seizure. Your veterinarian can help you with this, since the dosage must be determined by the dog's body weight and valium is a controlled substance and must be prescribed by a veterinarian. Keep an ice pack in the freezer. Any seizure lasting more than five minutes is considered serious and should be considered an emergency situation. Plan on how you will get your seizing dog to your car while having seizures. A make shift stretcher made from blankets or a plastic sheet will work. The dog can be carried or dragged depending on its size and number of people assisting. Call the animal hospital before you leave, and tell them you're coming. If it's late at night, some clinics lock their doors for security, and you can give them a heads up as to the medical situation.

7. **Relax** – Living with a dog with canine epilepsy or seizures at any time is very stressful for the caregiver. This stress can be harmful to the caregiver and the dog will notice your stress which will make your dog stressful too. Stress has other side effects also, like headaches, insomnia, aches, and pains. As the caregiver, you need to look at ways to destress. Talk to your doctor about ways to reduce your stress, preferably without drugs. Going for walks, or a run, exercise, talking to others, yoga, meditation are options together with many other healthy ways.

CHAPTER 33

Prognosis

The outlook for dogs with seizures ranges from a complete recovery, all the way to a grave fatal ending. This all depends on the cause of the condition. Primary epilepsy usually can be well-managed with oral anticonvulsants. Unfortunately, dogs with inoperable brain tumors or other brain lesions are at the other end of the prognostic spectrum.

Most forms of prevention will depend upon the frequency and underlying cause of the seizures. Your veterinarian may prescribe medications or, if there is a behavioral cause like loud surroundings, smoking, strong household cleaners, etc. that are the cause of seizures, you may be able to change the dogs environment to avoid such triggers.

Dietary management may also be recommended for small-breed puppies suffering from seizures due to hypoglycemia. These meals will typically consist of food that is high in protein, fat, and complex carbohydrates.

The ultimate goal in treating canine epilepsy is to restore a normal life for you and your epileptic dog through complete control of seizures with no side effects. However, this is frequently not possible and a more realistic goal would be to reduce the frequency and severity of the seizures without creating unacceptable side effects from the medications given. Usually even a well-controlled dog will have an occasional seizure.

Finding the right medication or combination of medications takes patience. Unfortunately, what works for one epileptic dog may not work for another. Medications need to be individualized to each specific dog's needs and this often requires trial and error to find the right medication and dose. Trying alternatives to medications with holistic or natural methods, you might find the break through you are looking for.

Good luck to you and your pet.

www.ingramcontent.com/pod-product-compliance
Lightning Source LLC
Chambersburg PA
CBHW020635220526
45464CB00001B/162